Training to be a physician

A Handbook of the Royal College of Physicians of London

Second edition

Compiled by the
Standing Committee of Members
of the Royal College of Physicians

1993

ROYAL COLLEGE OF PHYSICIANS OF LONDON

Royal College of Physicians of London
11 St Andrews Place, London NW1 4LE

Copyright © 1993 Royal College of Physicians of London
ISBN 1 873240 66 X

Typeset by Oxprint Limited, Aristotle Lane, Oxford
Printed in Great Britain by The Lavenham Press Ltd,
Lavenham, Sudbury, Suffolk.

Preface

Career guidance, organisation and prospects are all features of professional training often shrouded in clouds. In this book we aim to clear the clouds and reveal the geography, the potential routes and the information sources available for those embarking on the final ascent to the medical peak. If you are considering a post in medicine with a view to eventual consultant status, this series of articles holds invaluable information.

Medical training, practice and organisation are in the process of change and, as with early teenagers, it is not possible to predict their exact adult form. Some of the effects of *Achieving a balance** and the NHS reforms, with their subsequent subordination of education, are unpredictable, or at least unpredicted. Moreover, the European Community is introducing new regulations which are certain to affect the recognition of 'monospecialties' and the content and duration of their training programmes, and certification and accreditation as a specialist. The European Certificate represents a minimal period of specialty training sufficient to equip an independent specialist practising within the European Community, whereas a consultant in the NHS is not only an independent specialist but also has considerable administrative duties, including research and development in his clinical field, as well as the responsibility for training juniors.

If errors are found in the advice given in this book, the likelihood is that they can be attributed to unpredictability of developments at the time of writing. Nevertheless, as clear a view as is possible is presented and, where doubt exists, sources for further information are clearly identified.

The Members of the College, through their Standing Committee, have helped to produce this expanded second edition of *Training to be a physician*. We believe that it contains the information essential to all prospective physicians. We wish you all success in your future.

STANDING COMMITTEE OF MEMBERS
Royal College of Physicians
July 1993

Hospital Medical Staffing: Achieving a Balance—Plan for Action. London: Department of Health, 1987.

iii

Acknowledgements

We are grateful to the following for their contributions to the individual specialty sections:

Nick Beeching
Nicola Brain
Roger Briggs
John Catford
Kevin Channer
Dian Donnai
Gillian Ford
John Hodges
John Horsley
Nigel Hyman
Stanley Kaye
Ian Lewin
Ewan MacDonald
Neil Marlow
Lindsay McLellan
Alison Milne
Deborah Mitchell
Stephen Morgan
John Morrison

Fred Nye
Gilbert Park
Anthony Pinching
Anthony Redmond
Wynne Rees
Clive Roberts
Gillian Shepherd
Hilary Smith
Humberto Testa
Raj Thakker
Paul Tromans
Michael Tunbridge
Gillian Turner
Bob Walt
Sir David Weatherall
Ian Weller
Robin Winter
Ed Wraith

Contents

PART 1
Structures for training

1 Introduction

Since 1518 the primary function of the Royal College of Physicians of London has been to supervise and maintain high standards of medical practice. It also sets standards and conditions of training to ensure that doctors and specialists of the future will achieve these standards and continue to practise them at a time when medical knowledge and techniques are rapidly expanding whilst resources for patient care are disproportionately dwindling.

The Royal College of Physicians believes that not only adequate but also high quality training is vital for doctors intending to make a career as consultant physicians. It is fully aware that, at present, service commitments are often so heavy that doctors in training have little time or energy for study and that more formal supervised training is often deficient. Moreover, financial constraints often result in poor accommodation or learning resources. What does the College try to do to improve this?

Preregistration posts are supervised and monitored by the universities. Any problems connected with these posts should be discussed with the dean of the relevant medical school. Every senior house officer post and registrar post in medicine requiring approval for general professional training (Chapter 6) is inspected by a visiting team appointed by the College. Senior registrar posts and registrar posts considered suitable for higher medical training (Chapter 8) are assessed by a team appointed by the Joint Committee on Higher Medical Training.

The visiting teams review conditions of work and interview the doctors in post to hear their personal opinions. Posts are usually approved for five years but, where training conditions are deficient, a team will recommend approval for only a limited period to allow such deficiencies to be corrected. Explicit instructions and advice are given, but manpower shortage is often the crucial factor that creates inadequate conditions for training. Occasionally posts are not approved at all.

Doctors in training must have the opportunity to gain first-hand practical clinical experience. Service work is highly relevant, indeed essential, but it has to be properly supervised by senior doctors who must be readily available for consultation and discussion. Much of the stress under which junior doctors work is due to the fact that they often have to make life and death decisions with inadequate experience and without the guidance and support of a more senior doctor.

Senior doctors must accept that they have responsibilities for training their junior staff, not only in obvious ways such as help with diagnosis and treatment, but also in the equally important, less tangible aspects of the art and ethos of medicine. These include such things as the subtlety of patient–doctor partnerships; communication in a wide variety of circumstances needing tact, understanding and sensitivity; professional attitudes towards patients, towards paramedical staff and towards management. Indeed, high-quality professional attitudes must be nurtured in every facet of good doctoring if the consultants of the present and future are to contribute their best in their greatly privileged position of leading the team of all those involved in the care of patients.

MARGARET E. H. TURNER-WARWICK
President, Royal College of Physicians, 1989–92

2 The College's Role in Postgraduate Education

The College aims to educate doctors of all grades of seniority by acting as a forum where up-to-date and topical information and views are offered. It does not arrange courses specifically designed for postgraduate diploma examinations. The main thrust of the educational programme is clinical but, with increasing advances in technology and science, the educational programmes also emphasise basic science and its application to clinical practice. There are also conferences and courses to cover aspects of ethics, audit and management. Full information about these activities is available from the Conference Secretary at the College.

Teach-ins

The teach-ins are perhaps the most didactic of the College's teaching activities. Although not overtly planned as such, they are the closest the College comes to teaching specifically for the Membership examination. Selected topics, eg 'Update on peptic ulcer' and 'Problems with the treatment of asthma', are dealt with in detail. Each teach-in is arranged by a specialist in the field with a panel of expert speakers who give their views and form a brains trust for the audience's questions.

Many of the teach-ins have a chosen theme; following an overview there are sessions covering a number of topics linked with the overview. For example, the theme 'New aspects of metabolism as applied to clinical medicine' had specific sessions on diabetes, osteoporosis and neuropeptides.

In addition to the teach-ins in London, the College also holds three teach-ins per year, with a programme for a whole day, in regions outside London. They are arranged in conjunction with a local organiser and are intended for junior medical staff in all specialties. It is hoped that consultants will support this by releasing their juniors to attend the teach-in held in their region.

Conferences

The purpose of conferences is to present advances in medicine with an emphasis on the basic sciences as well as clinical aspects. There are three main types of conference.

Free ranging conferences

The Advanced Medicine Conference is a three- or four-day meeting, held each year in London. It covers a wide range of topics illustrating the impact of recent developments in clinical, laboratory and health services research on current clinical practice. Its proceedings are published as a book *Horizons in medicine.*

The annual Paediatric Conference is a two-day conference on single or multiple child health topics. Its proceedings are published in full by the College. There are also two-day regional conferences held in university medical schools outside London.

On a more futuristic note, the annual Science and Medicine Conference gives the audience the opportunity to hear eminent scientists present the most recent advances in their special areas of interest. Each session starts with a broad overview of the subject given by an expert in the field, followed by shorter talks by rising stars in science. The purpose of this meeting is to inform clinicians of the new thoughts and findings in the basic sciences which are likely to influence their clinical practice well into the next century. The College invites a number of medical students and junior medical staff to attend this conference as its guests.

Conferences on specific subjects

At these one- to three-day conferences a topic is explored and discussed in detail. Subjects range from those with wide general appeal, eg 'Assessing and assuring the quality of medical care' and 'Measurement of the outcome of medical interventions', to those of interest to more specialised groups of doctors, eg 'Gene therapy' and 'What to do in atheroma'. The College also holds conferences on administrative aspects of medicine, such as 'Medical training and the White Paper', 'Design, development and decline of a medicine' and 'The impact of the EC on medicine'.

One-day meetings

The College holds one-day meetings under the general heading 'Issues in medicine', designed to explore subjects which are controversial or about which there is indecision in the profession. These meetings are not to forge a consensus but simply to encourage debate. Both clinical and ethical subjects have been explored, eg 'Salt and hypertension' and 'Priorities in medical care'. More recently, stimulated by suggestions from the Standing Committee of Members and GPs with MRCP qualifications, the College has held three conferences on Interfaces in Medicine. These meetings aim to bring together GPs and hospital practitioners to discuss clinical problems that cross the boundary between community and hospital. Topics so far covered are cardiology, asthma, diabetes and rheumatology.

Courses

Courses entitled 'Getting the most out of management' are organised twice a year in conjunction with the King's Fund College, for up to 18 consultants per course. They deal with the wider issues of management not covered by the various regional courses that address topical and local issues. The programme is intended for consultants who have no or little previous experience in management but who want to be able to manage their service more effectively in the changing financial and organisational context of the NHS. The programme is not especially designed to meet the rather different needs of consultants who are clinical directors, serve as medical representatives on unit or district management boards, or are members of health authorities.

   Since 1987, two or three courses on AIDS have been held each year. Each course consists of lectures at the College and practical demonstrations at the major centres in London with particular experience of managing patients with HIV infection. A three-day course on aspects of nuclear medicine is also available, designed for those who intend to specialise in nuclear medicine or in other disciplines where nuclear medicine will form an important part of their practice.

Lectures

Each year the College presents 16 to 18 formal lectures, three or four of them at a regional centre. In some of these lectures the broad subject matter is stipulated in the endowment and their content usually reflects the special interest and experience of the invited lecturer. The College therefore has only partial control of the subject matter of these lectures. Although they usually accompany the conferences held throughout the year, they are an adjunct to, rather than an integral part of, the College's educational programme. Nonetheless, they present a rich and varied pool of information, history and review.

Some of the lectures are published with the conference proceedings, others in the *Journal* of the RCP.

Royal College of Physicians publications

The *Journal* of the RCP, published quarterly, presents a wide-ranging view of medicine for physicians of all interests. It also publishes original papers and material based on the College conferences and lectures to inform those who are unable to attend the meeting at the College. The College also publishes separate reports of working parties, conferences and guidelines for good practice, which cover a wide range of subjects of practical and ethical importance and concern; they are available on sale from the College.

Miscellaneous educational activities

The College holds weekly courses in French with a medical bias and a one-week residential course in France. It also administers a number of scholarships for travelling and for undertaking research work for two to three years.

Mindful of the problems some doctors have in relation to the Membership examination, there is a counselling service for those who are considered to need advice on the basis of their performance; this is, of course, also available to those who seek help themselves.

The College aims to provide a continual and varied diet of educational material which it attempts to keep topical, innovative and up to date in such a way that a physician of any age should find it stimulating and informative.

The Academic Registrar's office is always interested to receive suggestions for new conferences and courses.

3 The Role of the College Tutor

Where does the College tutor fit into the postgraduate medical education hierarchy? College tutors are appointed by and responsible to the Royal College of Physicians; their role includes:

- disseminating RCP information;
- organising and collating RCP surveys;
- arranging RCP visits for approval of posts for general professional training.

The clinical tutor, on the other hand, is responsible to the postgraduate dean and appointed by the local university. At unit level the clinical tutor has overall responsibility for *facilitation* of postgraduate educational activities across different specialties (Table 1).

The College appoints tutors throughout England and Wales. Their first task should be to advertise their existence; in many centres, junior hospital doctors do not even know who is the clinical tutor, let alone who is the RCP tutor who may also be responsible for aspects of their postgraduate education. Almost every medical unit (hospital) has a programme of postgraduate educational activities and the College tutor should ensure that his or her name appears on the front page of this programme alongside the names of the other 'specialty tutors' responsible to the other Royal colleges, eg surgery, psychiatry, radiology etc. The names of these 'specialty tutors' should also appear on a list in the postgraduate centre in each hospital, and should be readily available from the postgraduate secretary. If the name of the College tutor is not readily available, junior doctors should be encouraged to

Table 1. Postgraduate medical educational hierarchies

Royal College of Physicians	SCOPME (Standing Committee on Postgraduate Medical Education)	Other Royal colleges
Regional adviser	Regional postgraduate dean (university)	Regional advisers
College tutor	Clinical tutor	Other 'specialty' tutors

enquire from the local postgraduate secretary who the College tutor is and when he or she might be available to give advice.

Local postgraduate medical education committees

Most units now have a postgraduate education committee, which is chaired by the clinical tutor and should have, as members, specialty tutors responsible to all the Royal colleges. If appropriate, there may also be a representative of the undergraduate dean from the local university, at least one (preferably two) junior doctors, and a representative of management. In current changing times, with budgets for postgraduate education only recently set, it is vital that management, perhaps most appropriately from the personnel department, should be represented on this committee so that the full scope of postgraduate activities in a local hospital can be understood by management and, hopefully, supported with adequate funding.

Whom should a junior doctor consult?

Faced with a seeming embarrassment of riches in terms of people available to give postgraduate advice, it seems surprising that most junior doctors, when surveyed, say that there is no one to give them such advice. It is likely that this reflects the inadequate advertising of the existence of the postgraduate educational structure. Junior doctors should be encouraged, first and foremost, to seek advice and discuss problems with their own consultant who, in some circumstances, may also be their educational supervisor, although many districts have yet to appoint formal educational supervisors. More often than not, satisfactory advice can be obtained at this first port of call. However, in circumstances where further advice is required, there is a hierarchy that can be followed (Table 2). Where the problems relate to postgraduate medical education, for example in relation to the MRCP, the next person to consult should be the College tutor. If, however, the

Table 2. Hierarchy for a junior doctor to seek advice

1. Consultant (Educational supervisor)
2. College tutor
3. Clinical tutor
4. Regional adviser
5. Regional postgraduate dean

College tutor also happens to be the same person as the first person on the list, ie the junior doctor's own consultant, it is important that the registrar, SHO or house officer should know that the clinical tutor is also available for advice. If even that gives no satisfaction, the RCP regional adviser and/or the regional postgraduate dean can be consulted.

Needs of junior doctors

- *Counselling*. Many junior doctors, and perhaps some senior ones, do not appreciate the difference between counselling and career guidance. Counselling is a prospective, helpful activity that ideally all junior doctors ought to experience on a regular basis throughout their careers. Counselling entails identification of their strengths and weaknesses, and of their wants and needs. Many people perceive counselling to be remedial, implying something that happens only to failures, and to the 'stuck' doctor. However, getting stuck should be seen as a failure of the system; if regular prospective counselling had occurred, the doctor might not have become stuck, and certainly would not have been perceived as a failure. Prospective counselling should be the responsibility of the educational supervisor, but the College tutor in conjunction with the clinical tutor should be responsible for ensuring that it happens. They are therefore the organisers and facilitators of counselling, and the RCP tutor should play a major role in counselling juniors from medical specialties, as second in line in the hierarchy after the educational supervisor.

- *Career guidance*. Consultants think that career guidance happens routinely, yet SHOs will say that it does not. Again it is the College tutor's and the clinical tutor's responsibility to make career guidance available within the unit (local hospital). Most junior doctors should be advised to follow the hierarchy as set out in Table 2; however, one additional important source of information is, of course, their peer group. It is very important that they should also discuss careers not only with their SHO and registrar colleagues but also with senior registrars in the appropriate specialty.

- *MRCP examination advice*. Although this advice may also be sought from various sources within the local hospital, again perhaps following the hierarchy in Table 2, the College tutor is certainly the major source of information within the individual hospital. An SHO who is contemplating sitting the MRCP(UK) examination would do well to seek advice from the College tutor who can recommend the appropriate information published by the College about the examination, and would also be able to answer such questions as what it entails, when to do it, where to do it, and what is appropriate in the way of study leave or courses. The College tutor will have negotiated a local policy on leave with the clinical tutor who is responsible for signing study leave forms and, through the regional postgraduate dean, has access to the relevant budget. The College tutor is likely to be responsible, within the hospital, for organising MRCP teaching, which may be a locally run course or could be ward-based, and individual, or a combination.

General educational role of the College tutor

The precise extent of the role of the College tutor depends on whether or not the clinical tutor is also a physician. If the clinical tutor is not a physician, it will probably be the College tutor's responsibility to facilitate regular educational meetings, such as specific topic seminars, journal clubs, and weekly physicians' meetings (grand rounds). It is likely that the College tutor and the clinical tutor will discuss the integration of clinico-pathological meetings and audit, using both as educational tools. It may be that postgraduate (junior doctor) and continuing (consultant) medical education would be improved if it became more learner-centred. It is likely that the College tutor will be one of the clinical tutor's chief allies in exploring ways of changing our traditional teacher-centred methods of education and concentrating more on the needs of the learner.

Conclusion

The College tutor's role may have many ramifications but the education, counselling and guidance of the physician in training should be the pivot of his or her activities. From the College tutor's point of view, this is likely to be satisfying but time-consuming. Although education itself should be seen as part of the curriculum for a junior hospital doctor, and should be scheduled to happen between 9 am and 5 pm, it is likely that the College tutor's role will extend to evenings and weekends, or, to misquote Thomas à Kempis, *Sic transit gloria Sunday.*

4 The MRCP(UK) Examination

Evolution of the examination

The examination leading to the diploma MRCP(UK) evolved from the three separate and different examinations of the Royal College of Physicians of London, the Royal College of Physicians of Edinburgh and the Royal College of Physicians and Surgeons of Glasgow. It is organised through the Part 1 and Part 2 MRCP(UK) Boards whose Central Office is housed in the London college. Both boards have representatives of the three colleges and meet three times a year at each college in rotation. They are responsible to the joint committee of the three colleges, which meets twice yearly, and they also communicate directly with the body in each college concerned with the examination.

The first step in the evolution of the MRCP(UK) examination was the introduction in October 1968 of the common Part 1 multiple choice question (MCQ) paper. The same format of 60 MCQs, each with five completions, continues to the present day. However, to make it fairer for those intending to take Part 2 in paediatrics, from October 1993 Part 1 contains 50 per cent common core questions and 50 per cent with a bias towards paediatrics or adult medicine. On passing Part 1 there is an option to take Part 2 in either adult or paediatric medicine.

A common Part 2 paper set by the board was introduced in December 1972. The written papers are followed 5–6 weeks later by clinical and oral examinations of the same pattern though organised separately by each of the three colleges. Since September 1977 candidates have had the choice of sitting the whole of Part 2 in either general medicine or paediatrics. The successful candidates receive the same MRCP(UK) diploma without any differentiation being made between paediatrics and general medicine.

It was soon appreciated that candidates with marks lower than a bare fail in the written paper stood little or no chance of obtaining the additional marks required to compensate for this in the clinical and oral examinations. It was therefore decided that such candidates should not proceed with the examination (and should have their fee for the clinical and oral examinations refunded). By reducing the number of candidates taking the clinical and oral examinations, it became possible to extend the time allotted to the short case section of the clinical examination from 20 to 30 minutes. This ensures that every candidate can be examined in every major system of the body, and results in a much more rigorous and searching test. Other innovations have included testing candidates' cardiopulmonary resuscitation skills using artificial models.

Purpose of the examination

The MRCP(UK), unlike most other postgraduate medical diplomas, is an 'entry' rather than an 'exit' examination, for those intending to proceed to higher medical training. At the same time, by placing limits on attempts and time, it helps to redirect young doctors at a relatively early stage of their careers should they fail to achieve the standard required to commence training as potential consultant physicians or their equivalent. The colleges, through the Joint Committee on Higher Medical Training, play an important role in this further training by a system of inspection of training posts and accreditation of doctors who have completed approved training programmes.

The Part 1 MCQ paper is intended to test a broad range of theoretical knowledge with increasing emphasis on basic science as applied to clinical medicine. Part 2, in all its sections—written papers, clinicals and oral—tests the candidate's ability to apply the theoretical knowledge necessary to pass Part 1 to clinical situations and to show sound judgement in doing so. Part 2 should reflect good everyday clinical skills and practice as performed in the normal work situation.

Pass rate

Unlike an examination taken at the completion of training when most candidates would be expected to pass, the MRCP(UK) has a relatively low pass rate. With each Part 1 entry of 1,300–1,900 candidates, the board realises that the differences in the degree of difficulty of consecutive examinations inevitably are greater than differences in abilities of the large cohorts of candidates sitting each examination. A candidate's performance is assessed in relation to that of the other candidates (peer reference) rather than against an external standard of performance set by the examiners (criterion reference). As a result the pass mark (but not the pass rate) does vary at each examination.

A similar system is used in the Part 2 written paper examination, taken by up to 1,300 candidates three times a year. In the clinical and oral sections of the Part 2 examination, candidates are assessed as to whether they show the degree of competence required by the three pairs of examiners who assess them. The examiners know nothing of the candidate's performance in the written paper, or in previous attempts, and are thus using a criterion reference system. Notwithstanding this somewhat hybrid means of testing, the pass rate in Part 2 is also remarkably constant.

MRCP(UK) Part 1

The examination is held at 16 centres in the United Kingdom and 15 centres overseas. Candidates may enter 18 months after their date of graduation and are allowed up to four attempts.

The Part 1 examination is designed to assess a candidate's knowledge and understanding both of the basic sciences relevant to medical practice and of the common or important disorders, to a level appropriate for entry to specialist training.

The examination paper will cover elementary statistics, epidemiology and clinical sciences. Increased emphasis will in future be given to basic science topics. In both options, questions may be set on relevant principles of cell, molecular and membrane biology, immunology, genetics, and on biochemistry, as well as anatomical, physiological, microbiological and pharmacological topics.

Exclusively paediatric topics will no longer be tested in the section on general medicine. In the paediatric option a knowledge of embryology, fetal and child physiology, child and adolescent growth and development, and child and family psychology may also be tested.

One mark is awarded for a correct response (true or false) and one mark is deducted for an incorrect response; a zero mark is given to a 'don't know' answer. Each paper therefore has 300 marks to be earned from the 60 MCQs (each with five completions). Questions are submitted by examiners from all three colleges and by others with an interest in the examination. The Part 1 Board selects from the question bank a mixture of new and unused questions, revised bank questions and marker questions unchanged from previous use. The performance of candidates in the latter is of particular interest in trying to evaluate the increase (or decrease) in knowledge of cohorts of candidates of a particular subject over time and whether the standard of candidates in general is changing. Each board meeting also reviews the most recent examination. A statistical analysis is made of the performance of each question and each part of each question. Of particular value are:

- **The mean score** (the average of all the candidates' scores on a question, a measure of its *difficulty*) with a possible range from −1.0 to +1.0.
- **The correlation coefficient** between the score of each candidate on a question and his/her score in the examination as a whole, ie a measure of the *discriminatory power of the question as a whole*.
- **A further correlation coefficient** comparing the marks obtained in the examination as a whole of candidates who make a correct response to an individual item with those of candidates who make an incorrect response, ie a measure of the *discriminatory power of an individual item*.

With this information the board is able to modify questions, if necessary, before returning them to the bank.

The regulations allow candidates with certain qualifications from other colleges and bodies exemption from the MRCP(UK) Part 1.

MRCP(UK) Part 2

Having passed the MRCP(UK) Part 1 examination, the candidate is allowed a total of six attempts at the Part 2 examination which must be made within the next seven years. Entry is permitted after 2½ years training from the date of graduation, of which at least 12 months must be spent in posts involving the care of emergency medical patients after full registration with the General Medical Council. Up to three attempts may be made through one college, two through one of the other colleges, plus one attempt through the third college.

The whole Part 2 examination is held only in the United Kingdom and Hong Kong (restricted to doctors working there). The written section alone is held in a few overseas centres, with successful candidates coming to the UK to complete the examination.

The written section has three separate parts: case history, data interpretation and photographic material. Each part contributes equally to the final score which means that it is not necessary to pass each part provided the total mark reaches the required pass mark. Unlike Part 1, the marks are awarded on a sliding scale, each question, or a small group of questions, being marked by a scoring group in one of the three colleges. The colleges take it in turn to mark one whole paper, so a scoring group of 4–6 examiners will mark every candidate answering a particular question. This gives them considerable insight into the performance of that question in the examination. The scoring group works to an answer key, devised by the board at the time of setting the question, which tries to anticipate the various answers candidates might give; there are no negative marks in Part 2. The scoring group is allowed to make alterations and additions to the proposed answer key to allow for unanticipated answers, and also to revalue the proposed marks provided it does not alter the maximum mark obtainable for a question. Each scoring group submits a report to the Part 2 Board of its experience in marking the question with recommendations as to how that question might be improved. When the board reviews the written section, additional statistical information will be available similar to that in Part 1. The mean mark of all candidates for a particular question is a measure of its difficulty. A correlation coefficient compares the performance of candidates in a particular question with their performance in the paper as a whole, this being a measure of the discriminatory power of a question. With the above strands of information and advice, the Part 2 Board can then modify stem questions or answers appropriately before returning them to the bank.

Potential questions for the examination are submitted by examiners and others to any of their three colleges. Each college has question groups in general medicine and paediatrics who process and edit the questions and pass them on to the Central Office.

The clinical and oral examinations are organised by the individual colleges but follow the pattern laid down by the Part 2 Board. To help achieve, as far as is possible, uniformity in examining standards, one of the six examiners who make up the three pairs will be from one of the other two colleges. Examiners are briefed by a senior examiner before each examination, and a final meeting of examiners is held to review the results.

Examiners are asked to write comments assessing the various attributes of candidates and their performance. Candidates who have failed particularly badly are counselled by their sponsor or College tutor and may be advised to defer their next entry by one examination if it is felt that they would benefit from further training and practice. Other candidates may also be offered or given counselling, if requested by them or one of their sponsors.

The performance of examiners is also assessed by comparing the marks they award in the different sections throughout the examination with those of their peers, to achieve a 'hawk-dove' index.

Further details regarding the MRCP(UK) can be found in the

following publications of the three Royal colleges and obtainable from them:

MRCP(UK) Examination Regulations (free)
MRCP(UK) Part 1 Papers (1991) (£6.00)
MRCP(UK) Part 1 Paediatric Option: specimen paper (£2.00)
MRCP(UK) Part 2 Papers (1986) (£10.00)

5 The Role of the Regional Adviser

Regional adviser posts were created in response to the effective organisation of the National Health Service on a regional basis in 1969 and were intended to establish a College presence outside London. As the work gradually increased, deputies were appointed, so now each region has an adviser and a deputy. Both are practising physicians; one is usually recruited from a district with a teaching hospital and the other from a district without one.

Advisers are appointed to the regions in England, Wales and Northern Ireland and there are also advisers overseas. There are no such posts in Scotland, which has Royal colleges in Edinburgh and Glasgow.

The usual method of appointment is for the Fellows in each region to elect a deputy adviser who succeeds the adviser after two to three years.

Regional advisers in paediatrics

Regional advisers in paediatrics carry out precisely the same role in relation to paediatrics as do regional advisers in adult specialties.

Main activities

Details of the wide-ranging role of regional advisers are given below.

Liaison with Fellows and Members in the region

The regional adviser, who can be consulted by any Member or Fellow in the region, also maintains close contact with the College tutors in order to keep Fellows, Members and others in the region informed of College policy and actions and, in turn, brings to the College regional opinion, ideas, doubts, suggestions and criticisms. In larger regions such consultations may be shared with the deputy regional adviser.

Meetings of regional advisers

The advisers and deputies meet quarterly at the College. The meeting is chaired by the President; the College officers and representatives of the Censors and Council also attend. Any regional adviser can add any subject to the agenda that needs to be discussed. Although the function of the meeting is advisory only, its influence is considerable.

Membership of regional specialist subcommittees

The subcommittee gives the consultants of each specialty the opportunity to discuss common policy and to inform and advise the regional medical officer. The advisers are *ex officio* members of the regional specialist subcommittees which usually meet twice a year. The place of the meeting may change, giving opportunities to visit various hospitals and districts within the region. Although the advisers are full members of each of the committees, their main responsibilities are to listen to the problems that concern the College and try to interpret College recommendations and views. The advisers have direct access to the regional medical officers and officers of the regional health authority. With the current changes in organisation, advisers' opinions on regional problems are frequently sought.

Consultant appointments

The College selects one of its Fellows to serve as the College representative on appointments committees for consultants in medical specialties. Before a consultant post is advertised, it must be approved by the regional adviser, who is responsible for assessing all aspects of the proposed job, particularly the facilities available and junior staff support. He or she may seek the opinion of other Fellows, usually the chairman of the appropriate regional specialist group or subcommittee.

Senior registrar appointments

The advisers are also involved in the appointment of senior registrars in medical specialties. There is no formal representation of the College on these statutory committees but most regions ask the regional adviser to nominate a representative. The regional adviser may be the representative but, if the subject is outside the adviser's specialty, he or she will usually nominate another Fellow within the region to represent the College.

Registrar appointments

Since the introduction of career registrars and the transfer of contracts to the regions, the regional adviser or a College representative sits on appointments committees.

Nominations for Fellowship and distinction awards

Members of the College may be nominated for the Fellowship once a year, the closing date being 1st November. Soon after this date the advisers receive the list of nominations for their regions. They make enquiries among the Fellows to determine the support for these nominations and then transmit their findings to the College. The advisers are not involved in making the final decisions. The College is asked to propose its Fellows and Members for distinction awards and one of the advisers attends the College 'C' awards committee. They take soundings in the region before the meeting of the committee. They do not attend the higher awards committee but may suggest names.

Professional training

The advisers are involved in the assessment of posts for recognition for general professional training. They are thus concerned in the approval of senior house officer posts and most registrar posts, which must be so approved before they are advertised.

The Training Office in the College maintains a list of recognised posts which is circulated to advisers to ensure that re-assessment by a visit takes place when recognition is about to lapse, usually after five years. The visit may be conducted by the regional adviser and/or the deputy adviser, together with the paediatric adviser. Every ten years visits are conducted by assessors from outside the region. In liaison with the postgraduate dean, the advisers monitor the recommendations of the visiting team, the visit being organised by the College tutor in collaboration with the clinical tutor and local clinicians. The advisers are not responsible for approval of posts for higher medical training which is organised directly by the JCHMT, although they may be members of a visiting team.

Other activities

The advisers are *ex officio* members of the regional postgraduate committee and as such may serve on its subcommittees. They are frequently concerned with the training facilities for junior staff. They may be asked by the College to counsel candidates who have difficulty in passing the MRCP examination and give advice on career prospects.

The regional advisers are at times involved in the collection of information for the College. This has included the on-take commitment of general physicians, the organisation of ethics committees and the establishment of registrar and research posts. In conjunction with the district College tutors they are responsible for encouraging appropriate audit activities in each district.

Conclusion

The creation of the post of regional adviser to establish a College presence outside London has been successful, as can be seen by the increase in work and responsibilities, and has led to the appointment of College tutors.

The activities of the advisers have resulted in Fellows and Members of the College and other members of the medical profession and health service managers becoming increasingly aware of the wide function and responsibility of the Royal College of Physicians.

6 Consultant Appointments Committees

Appointment of a consultant in the National Health Service follows a set procedure: the appointment must be advertised, an advisory appointments committee (AAC) must be convened, an interview held and the person selected by the committee recommended to the regional health authority. In the case of academic appointments (eg senior lecturers) the College is usually, but not obligatorily, invited to send a representative to the appointments committee.

Before a post can be advertised, several steps must be taken. The district health authority or, where applicable, the hospital trust decides the nature of the appointment it would like to see made. Whether it is a new post or a replacement, there may be conflicting views on its character and on details of the job description. Local medical opinion is likely to predominate in making the decisions, but the administration will also have its say.

When the appropriate authority has decided what it wants, but before the post can be advertised, the job description is submitted for approval by the regional adviser, who may ask that certain aspects be changed or, rarely, even disallow the appointment altogether. The regional adviser may take advice concerning a proposed appointment from officers of the regional specialty committee and/or the chairman or secretary of the College specialty committee. College committees in the various specialties have drawn up guidelines to help regional advisers assess the suitability of an appointment, giving general guidance as to the facilities and resources required for a consultant appointment in that specialty. These guidelines have been scrutinised by the Council of the College to make sure that they are in harmony with each other and that, while insisting on essential requirements, they do not demand so much that the post becomes impossibly expensive. It should be noted that it is the clear view of the Royal College of Physicians that accreditation is *not* a requirement for appointment as a consultant.

When its description has been approved, the post is advertised in the medical press. A consultant AAC for that post is set up. Its composition is determined by statute and includes two representatives from the district authority (usually doctors from the hospital where the appointment is to be made), and at least one colleague from the same specialty, a teaching hospital representative and a College representative (CR). The CR, who must come from outside the NHS region concerned, is almost invariably a fairly senior Fellow of the College. Most Fellows are regarded as suitable to represent the College on consultant AACs but some may be less so, perhaps because of their narrow field of interest or because they are known to have many other commitments. The College tries to ensure that a wide variety of Fellows represents it on these important committees.

Methods of short-listing vary; the CR should be fully involved in this process. The commonest method is for each member of the committee to mark the candidates and then four or five are invited for interview.

The CR is a full member of the AAC, with neither more nor less power than the others, and is charged by the College with seeing that the selected candidate is adequately trained for the appointment, but this does not mean that the candidate must be accredited; indeed, CRs are specifically asked to be flexible on this point. If a candidate is appropriate for the appointment but lacks some limited aspect of training, for example proficiency in a technique, the AAC may recommend that he or she undertakes further training for a few weeks or months before taking up the appointment. The recommendation of the committee is usually announced to the candidates at the end of the meeting.

The CR is free to question applicants on all aspects of their application, not merely the adequacy or otherwise of their specialist experience. The CR is asked by the College to emphasise its interest in encouraging research and to bring out a candidate's research contributions. The CR has a vote in the committee's decision but does not have a veto; if not satisfied about a selection, the CR may report to the College and even, exceptionally, ask the College to take up the objections with the regional health authority.

The number and quality of applicants for consultant appointments vary greatly. Some specialties are less popular than others and may attract few and poor applications; occasionally for this reason no appointment is made. In other specialties the pressure is intense and 10–20 high-class applications may be received.

7 Advice on Applying for Consultant Appointments

Members often raise questions about the 'fairness' of advisory appointments committees for NHS consultant posts. It is therefore appropriate to include a personal view on a sensible approach to the ordeal of applying for a permanent job.

The job description for a consultant post will usually have been carefully drawn up to suit the needs of the department concerned but is also influenced by other senior hospital staff and, increasingly, by district managers. So statements such as 'A special interest would be an advantage' require further informal investigation. The department might have clear ideas as to what that special interest should be but have been prevented from making the job description too specific; similarly, the job description may have been designed to suit a candidate known to other members of the department, though this may not be immediately obvious. Careful, even probing, enquiries may be needed to establish how your prospective colleagues and administrators envisage your pattern of work and interests, so that this discovery is not made at a wasted interview and to guard against being appointed to a job that is not as you had expected it to be. A visit to the district to make tactful enquiries is an important initial mutual assessment between applicant and potential colleagues. This has to include a discussion with the business manager about the trust's or provider unit's plans, the purchaser's aims and any effects of local financial pressure and future service developments. It is also important at this stage to clarify junior staff allocation, their hours of work, split rotas etc.

An application should always be accompanied by a clear statement of why you want the job, what you hope to contribute to the hospital, and stress the appropriateness of your qualifications and experience. Weighting your *curriculum vitae* is entirely appropriate—all of your training will not be equally applicable to the rest of your professional life; for example, research experience would probably need different emphasis in applications for a teaching hospital and a DGH post. But always be scrupulously honest in your statements. Word processors are invaluable!

During the period after applying, most appropriately after being short-listed, it is important to give your future colleagues and administrators the opportunity of getting to know you, at least superficially, and vice versa. The appointment of a close colleague is one of the most important professional decisions of a lifetime and has to be likened to a marriage. It is not in the interests of either party to appoint an incompatible colleague and, while no member of the committee has a veto, a statement by the department representative that a particular candidate would be difficult to work with would be a high hurdle to jump at the interview. In this context the question of favouring a local or known candidate can be put in perspective. 'The devil you know' is a powerful argument. In spite of this it is rare for an advisory appointments committee's decision to be a foregone conclusion, particularly if the job has attracted a good field. It is unwise to withdraw because you know there is a strong local candidate; in the first place, all is not always as it appears from outside; second, strong support in favour of a candidate from an individual member of the committee who knows him or her (and will have declared this) is unlikely to have a major effect on the outcome; finally, the feared rival candidate may withdraw or be appointed elsewhere before the interview.

If, after your enquiries, you decide that you really want the post and appear to be appropriately qualified, it is clearly necessary to examine your own strengths and weaknesses (particularly those that you inappropriately included or omitted from your application). You will need to be prepared to defend (or acknowledge and explain) the latter, preferably with suggestions as to how they might be remedied before taking up the appointment.

At the interview it is rarely the *curriculum vitae* that decides the recommendation of the committee. Honesty and openness are important—probing questions are usually probing for a good reason, and it is unusual for the committee to be deceived. Personality is an important consideration but you will not be marked down for an expected degree of nervousness. Clear statements as to your aims and ambitions in the new post are valuable—most committees wish to feel that you know where you are going, and that you will pay due attention to the needs and aspirations of your future colleagues.

Given that more than one candidate with appropriate qualifications and experience appears at the interview, factors other than those on the application form will probably decide the outcome. To complain 'I was better qualified for the job' (than the person appointed) is to a great extent irrelevant; if the appointed candidate was less qualified on his *curriculum vitae* it is necessary to examine other qualities which you perhaps lacked at that interview.

It is rare for the recommendation of an AAC to be unfair; it is more usual for apparent unfairness to be due to the committee having given weight to less obvious attributes of the candidates. The role of the College's representatives on the advisory appointments committees is outlined in Chapter 6.

8 Postgraduate Training

Until 1953 there was no obligation for recently qualified doctors to undertake any further training before being admitted to the medical register maintained by the General Medical Council. It was on the recommendation of the Goodenough Committee on Medical Schools, which reported in 1944,[1] that the preregistration year of internship was introduced. Under the Medical Act of 1950 it became compulsory for every doctor after passing the qualifying examination to spend a period as a resident in an approved hospital before becoming eligible to proceed to full registration. This provision came into force on 1st January 1953. In 1964 the Royal College of Physicians published its *Report on training for consultants*[2] which suggested that, after becoming fully registered, those aspiring to a consultant career in a medical specialty should spend a further three years in general professional training followed by four years in the chosen specialty. However, as the result of continuing discussions and harmonisation of European Community regulations, it is likely that it will become possible to be recognised as a specialist physician after a shorter period of training.

The report of the Royal Commission on Medical Education (the Todd report, 1968)[3] recommended that the preregistration year should be followed by a structured programme of postgraduate training.

General professional training

The requirements considered to be desirable for general professional training (GPT) were defined in the first report of the Joint Committee on Higher Medical Training:[4]

> GPT will ordinarily occupy a period of three years after registration. Such training will be obtained in posts approved for this purpose providing general medical care, with or without 'special experience and training' in certain specialties. A proportion of this time may be spent in general practice under conditions approved for training purposes. Rigidity in training programmes will be avoided, subject to the suggested restrictions on time to be spent in certain types of posts. Trainees may rotate during GPT, possibly part time, through other specialties related

28

> to medicine such as clinical pathology, psychiatry and paediatrics. The candidate who has completed GPT should be 'pluripotential' in the sense that the training by its nature has not committed the doctor to continuing in a special branch of medicine.

This definition offers scope for a broad choice of educational opportunity but difficulties have arisen because of the limited availability of SHO posts in the more popular subjects and the tendency of some specialties to encourage their recruits to enter the specialty too early. An additional factor has been the advent of vocational training schemes for general practice which incorporate many posts in the popular specialties and so limit the availability of these posts for others.

Approval of posts

All junior hospital posts require educational approval if they are to be filled by doctors in training. Since the standards required by the Royal College of Physicians for GPT and those for vocational training for general practice by the Royal College of General Practitioners are so similar, a system of joint approval by both colleges has been established, hospital visits being carried out by teams with representatives from each college.

The Linacre Fellow of the College has a special responsibility for the approval of posts for GPT and, through the Training Office of the College, works closely with regional advisers and College tutors to ensure that posts are inspected or reviewed at the appropriate time. Hospitals are required to submit individual specialty forms in respect of newly established posts and in respect of any established posts being restructured or due for review. The visiting team normally consists of two physicians nominated by the Royal College of Physicians (one of whom is chairman), a paediatrician when paediatric posts are being inspected, and a representative of the Royal College of General Practitioners. The district College tutor makes the detailed arrangements for the visits in collaboration with the regional adviser and the regional adviser in paediatrics, and can provide valuable information about local conditions.

During visits the team will meet the consultants for a general discussion about the work of the hospital and will enquire about the educational facilities and training programmes. Specific questions will be asked about the laboratory and radiology services available, and the postgraduate centre and medical library will be visited. The SHOs and registrars will then be interviewed individually and confidentially, when their clinical duties and weekly teaching activities will be discussed. It is important for them to understand that it is the posts that are being assessed and not they themselves. The visiting team will wish to be assured that trainees are only asked to accept responsibility appropriate for their experience, that their work is adequately supervised and that they have access to advice from senior staff whenever necessary. It will also ask about the ways in which the work of the unit concerned is reviewed and assessed and whether the unit undertakes any form of regular audit.

The Linacre Fellow submits the reports of visiting teams to a subcommittee of the College Committee on General (Internal) Medicine which confirms or modifies the recommendations of the visitors. Final approval of posts for general professional training is granted by Comitia.

Difficulties have arisen in the past over the approval for general professional training of SHO or registrar posts in specialist departments. This has applied to posts in departments of cardiology, dermatology and genito-urinary medicine, and also to certain paediatric posts. However, it is recognised that experience in specialist departments may be beneficial, and it is now agreed that it is on its educational value that the suitability of a post for GPT should be judged. Nevertheless, although entirely suitable for those aspiring to a hospital career, some specialist posts may not be suitable for vocational training for general practice.

MRCP(UK) examination

All those who intend to make a career in hospital medicine require the MRCP which must be obtained before entering higher professional training. Candidates for Part 1 of the examination must have completed 18 months training since qualification. Candidates for Part 2 must have completed 18 months since full registration. No posts are specifically approved for the MRCP but candidates must have spent 12 months in posts involving the care of acutely ill medical patients, either adults or children, and are required to submit evidence that they have done so. The immediate objective for individuals completing the pre-registration year and contemplating a career in a medical specialty must therefore be a series of good posts at SHO level, arranged individually or as a rotation, to provide experience that will prepare them for this examination.

Career advice

During the period of GPT, trainees will aim to identify the specialty that they ultimately wish to follow. Regional postgraduate deans and district clinical tutors are the official sources of career advice and should have appropriate information available in their offices. Regional advisers and College tutors will also help. Consultants should always be willing and usually able to advise their juniors but it seems that most doctors in training seek information from their immediate seniors on the training ladder. The serious imbalance between numbers of training posts and career posts will eventually be corrected, and an increase in the number of consultants has long been agreed to be necessary.

The present situation makes it imperative for young doctors planning a career in hospital medicine to take full advantage of the posts available for general professional training, to remain 'pluripotential' for as long as possible and to take advantage of opportunities that may arise for higher professional training, though not necessarily in the specialty of their first choice.

Higher medical training

Training for a specialty in most branches of British medicine has always been arduous, and the ultimate objective of obtaining a consultant post has often been difficult to achieve.

This difficulty is in some respects a measure of the high standard and competitive nature of specialist practice in Britain; in other respects it is a manifestation of an unsatisfactory career structure which in recent years has been characterised by a serious imbalance between the numbers of training posts and career posts. In some specialties this imbalance at senior registrar level has been corrected, the number of senior registrar posts being closely related to the anticipated vacancies at consultant level. However, at the time of publication of this book there are still nearly three times as many registrars as would be required to fill the vacancies anticipated in the senior registrar grade. The Short report[5] recommended a reduction in the number of registrars and an increase in the number of consultants, with a shift from a 'consultant led' to a 'consultant provided' hospital service. The profession has agreed in principle to the proposals, as long as no reduction in junior staff takes place without a compensatory increase in consultant staff. Progress in this matter has been slow but the Joint Planning Advisory Committee (1985) made recommendations on senior registrar numbers, and proposals for bringing registrar numbers into balance with those of senior registrars were published in 1986 in the report *Achieving a balance*. These proposals involved a drastic reduction in the number of registrar posts available for UK graduates, but definitive numbers have not yet been agreed. Any registrar aspiring to a specialist career would be wise to ascertain the career prospects in the intended specialty by closely examining the ratios of career registrars to SRs and of SRs to consultants, as well as the average length of time spent by SRs in different medical specialties. He/she should also discuss possible changes in these figures with a senior member of the specialty before embarking on a particular career path.

Joint Committee on Higher Medical Training (JCHMT)

Those planning a career in a medical specialty must obtain an appointment to a post approved for higher medical training by the JCHMT. Hitherto such posts were at senior registrar level, but registrar posts considered to be providing higher training may now be approved.

The JCHMT was set up in 1970 as the result of consultations between the three Royal Colleges of Physicians (Edinburgh, Ireland and London), the Royal College of Physicians and Surgeons of Glasgow and members of the Association of Professorial Heads of Academic Departments of Medicine and Paediatrics. The responsibilities of the committee are 'to formulate guidelines for training in medical specialties, to approve posts and training programmes which are suitable for higher medical training and to grant certificates of accreditation to those who have completed higher medical training'.

Thus the JCHMT now plays an active part in co-ordinating higher training in all the medical specialties. The assessment and review of senior registrar posts are carried out by visiting teams set up by the appropriate specialist advisory committee (see below). The normal period of approval for established NHS senior registrar and university lecturer posts is five years. In the case of certain research posts, educational approval will be granted on an *ad personam* basis for the tenure of the incumbent concerned.

The JCHMT publishes a training handbook (the 'blue book')[6] which can be obtained from the Training Office of the Royal College of Physicians of London. It offers valuable information about the training requirements for each specialty, the composition of the committee and the names and addresses of all the postgraduate deans in the UK.

Specialist advisory committees

Specialist advisory committees (SACs) were established within the JCHMT to determine the training programmes for individual specialties. There are 22 such SACs with normally six members each, three being nominated by the JCHMT on recommendation by the four Royal colleges, the other three being nominated by the appropriate specialist association. (Variations in the composition of SACs are indicated in the training handbook.)

Every effort is made to ensure that the membership of SACs is well balanced, with adequate representation of universities and academic departments, regional physicians and younger consultants. Some regard for geographical 'spread' is also desirable. The tenure of membership of SACs is normally four years and each committee elects its own chairman.

Enrolment

On appointment to a substantive senior registrar or registrar post (NHS or honorary) approved for higher training, trainees should apply to the JCHMT for enrolment for higher training in the specialty or specialties concerned. Enrolment forms can be obtained from postgraduate deans and from the JCHMT office in the College.

Eligibility for enrolment will depend on having completed the required period of general professional training and obtained the MRCP(UK) or equivalent qualification. Retrospective recognition may be sought for relevant experience gained after completion of general professional training and obtaining the MRCP(UK). The SAC will indicate what period of post-Membership training is considered suitable for retrospective recognition towards higher training. The maximum period of retrospective recognition that may be granted is 24 months for single specialty accreditation and 12 months in each subject for dual accreditation.

Accreditation

The granting of accreditation signifies that the trainee has satisfactorily completed the prescribed period of higher training in the specialty or specialties concerned. However, the advisory appointments committee determines the suitability of a candidate for appointment to a specific consultant post and accreditation is not an obligatory requirement. At the same time it is likely that the majority of successful applicants will have been accredited in the specialty concerned.

Trainees should apply for accreditation towards the end of their higher medical training programme, taking into account any period of retrospective recognition. The award of a certificate of accreditation as recognition of completion of higher medical training is currently under review in the light of European Community directives.* The forms obtainable from the JCHMT office should be signed by the postgraduate dean and one of the supervising consultants, and submitted to the JCHMT office.

Overseas experience

The JCHMT recognises the value of overseas experience, but for accreditation applicants must have had a minimum of two years training at senior registrar level in the UK in approved posts. Trainees should seek the advice of the JCHMT about such periods of training well in advance of departure. They may also be asked to supply documentation of overseas training when applying for enrolment or accreditation. However, it is not always possible to offer prospective recognition of a proposed period of overseas training.

Research experience

The JCHMT recognises that participation in research forms an important part of training. In the case of single specialty accreditation, up to two years of relevant research, not necessarily involving clinical responsibilities for patients, may be accreditable.

Flexibility

The objective of the JCHMT is to improve and maintain standards of training. The SACs give considerable thought and care to ensure that the training programmes are comprehensive and relevant to the specialty, and appreciate that they need to pursue a policy of flexibility when considering the training of individuals seeking accreditation. SACs are constantly reminded that they must not practise rigidity while preaching flexibility.

Unusual training programmes — *ad hoc* committee

It is recognised that some trainees may follow training programmes that do not fall within the purview of any of the existing SACs and cannot reasonably be considered by the established procedure for approval of training for dual or triple accreditation. An *ad hoc* committee was established with a core membership of the chairman of the JCHMT, the medical co-ordinator and the chairman of the SAC in

*See note added in proof, page 48.

general (internal) medicine. The committee co-opts appropriate additional members as necessary. This committee considers requests for approval of unusual training programmes and subsequent accreditation for those who may have followed such programmes. Applications for approval of specialist training programmes, or accreditation, in unusual fields should be addressed to the medical co-ordinator, who will determine whether the request is appropriate for the *ad hoc* committee.

Career guidance

It is hoped that senior registrars will establish good working and personal relationships with their supervising consultants who will normally be their main source of advice. They should be able to help with the publication of scientific papers and the preparation of theses and, when the time comes, should be willing to advise their senior registrars on applying for consultant posts. Advice on the preparation of a *curriculum vitae* and on interview technique may be helpful at this stage.

Each regional health authority has a senior registrar training committee which oversees the progress of senior registrars in the region. The postgraduate dean and the College regional adviser are both members of this committee and they will be available for advice if necessary.

Finally, although it is not normally the function of the JCHMT to offer career advice, the Linacre Fellow, who acts as medical co-ordinator for the JCHMT, will be glad to respond to any specific queries concerning training programmes and matters relating to accreditation.

References

1. *Report of the Interdepartmental Committee on Medical Schools* (the Goodenough Committee) (1944). London: HMSO.
2. Royal College of Physicians (1964). *Report on Training for Consultants.*
3. *Report of the Royal Commission on Medical Education, 1965–68* (1968). London: HMSO.
4. *First Report of the Joint Committee on Higher Medical Training*, October 1972.
5. Social Services Committee (1980–81) *Fourth Report: Medical Education*. London: HMSO.
6. Joint Committee on Higher Medical Training (1990/91) *Training Handbook*. London: Royal College of Physicians.

9 Part-time Training

Although far from easy, it is permissible to undertake any or all of training on a part-time basis, provided the trainee undertakes not less than five weekly sessions and obtains some regular out-of-hours on-call experience. A session is normally defined as a standard unit of medical time (UMT) and will normally be four hours between the weekday hours of 9 am and 5 pm. Someone training for 5 UMTs a week would be expected to undertake half as much on-call work as someone training full-time (10 UMTs).*

Preregistration posts

The General Medical Council permits half-time training to be spread over two years. This can be arranged by the subdean of a medical school and can take the form of job sharing or be in a specially created post.

General professional training

At present there are no manpower restrictions on part-time SHO posts. District health authorities can create posts in response to demand, although it requires a great deal of persistence and determination to convince medical personnel officers that this can be done. It is important that these posts be approved by the College regional adviser as educationally appropriate. A combination of financial stringency and blinkered thinking has meant that less than 1% of SHOs are currently training on a part-time basis, despite the absence of manpower constraints at this level.

Professional training

Registrar level

In accordance with the plan for action that followed the national agreement *Achieving a balance*, training at registrar level is regarded as part of higher professional training. In January 1991 the NHS

*See note added in proof, page 39.

Management Executive, acting on the advice of the Joint Planning Advisory Committee (JPAC), issued an executive letter, EL(91)5, to each region in England and Wales, agreeing part-time career registrar quotas by specialty group. These posts are at present funded by the Department of Health, whereas existing part-time registrar posts are funded by the authority that holds the contract, ie the regional health authority or special health authority, or by the district health authority. Part-time career registrar posts are being advertised and filled by open competition, as are full-time career registrar posts. An additional reserve of posts is available for bids from special health authorities or from regional health authorities that have exceeded their quota, and these too are centrally funded. Regional and special health authorities are permitted to increase their part-time posts by dividing existing career registrar posts in two, provided there is local agreement. These posts do not receive central funding.

Health authorities are empowered to make a number of appointments of part-time visiting registrars for doctors who have come to the UK for up to four years of postgraduate training from outside the European Community since 1st April 1985. These posts cannot be used for UK graduates, doctors in the European Community and doctors who were in the UK before 1st April 1985.

Senior registrar level (the PM(79)3 scheme)

Each year the Department of Health, on the advice of the JPAC, releases a limited number of part-time senior registrar posts in each specialty. An advertisement inviting applications from suitably trained men or women who are prevented from working full-time for well founded personal reasons appears in the medical journals in August and September. Applicants can obtain forms from the Department of Health and seek interviews with their postgraduate dean to discuss their career plans and training needs. The next step in all but the smaller specialties is for a national assessment committee to be set up in one of the regions. These committees are constituted in the same format as full-time senior registrar appointment committees, and they act in a similar way, shortlisting candidates and calling for interview those considered most suitable for training at this level. Candidates in specialties where there are very few applicants may be referred for assessment to a full-time senior registrar appointment committee already meeting in one of the regions. These interviews usually take place in the winter following the national advertisement.

Successful candidates must then request the region in which they live to create and fund personal posts for them by approaching the regional consultant in public health medicine with responsibility for medical staffing. They must also find a suitable place to undertake training and, acting on advice from their postgraduate dean or the College regional specialty adviser, prepare a training programme and get it approved by the Joint Committee on Higher Medical Training. As for part-time registrar posts, these part-time senior registrar posts must include on-call duties.

Once the training programme is approved, the region will set up a local appointment committee to make sure that the candidate is suitable for the post that is being created. Unsuccessful candidates will be notified and encouraged to find out why they failed from either the postgraduate dean or the consultant in public health medicine (medical staffing) so that they can take remedial action before applying the following year.

Applicants for part-time training can also apply for full-time posts in the normal way. Part-time senior registrars can apply to their public health consultant to increase their sessions if circumstances change. Regions vary in the degree of flexibility on the number of sessions they will approve and fund.

If a senior registrar in part-time training moves to another region, the manpower approval moves with that individual. The new region must be asked to fund a part-time post, and the senior registrar will need to consult and prepare a training programme and get approval of it from the JCHMT.

Doctors who have already obtained a full-time senior registrar post in open competition need not apply under the national competition, nor need they appear before a local interviewing committee. They should approach the consultant in public health medicine (medical staffing) for a funded part-time post and prepare and obtain Joint Committee approval for a training programme.

Job sharing

In theory it is possible to train as an SHO, registrar or senior registrar by sharing a post with another person at a similar level of training. The practical difficulties are considerable — the job sharer must be found and must agree to undertake his or her half of the duties each week in the same specialty and at the same unit. Appointment committees take some convincing that two post-holders will be better than one. Those who have employed two job sharers are generally enthusiastic as they have experienced the benefits and found that most half-time trainees give considerably more than half-time to their work. Before participating in a job-sharing scheme, the contractual arrangements for annual, sick, maternity and study leave and superannuation should be clarified. The employing authority should be asked to confirm its intention to continue employing one of the job sharers even if the other moves away.

Drawbacks to part-time training

There are certain drawbacks to part-time training. The arrangements are complex and the procedures for obtaining a suitable training post and obtaining educational approval are extremely protracted. Funding often proves an insuperable difficulty. Ageism is rife in the medical profession and, since the relevant advisory committees expect those training on a part-time basis to spend twice as many years as those training full-time, part-time training for any lengthy period is not to be recommended if it is unlikely to be completed before the age of forty. Because training may take twice as long, the trainee is particularly vulnerable to changes in educational requirements. It is advisable to check with College tutors that requirements have not been changed, either by a change in policy or because of the impact of increased specialisation and a demand for additional higher qualifications. The final drawback is the entrenched attitude of many older consultants to any training that is less than full-time. This is particularly marked on oversubscribed specialties where the part-time trainee has traditionally been regarded as someone pursuing a soft option.

Non-training posts

It is possible to gain experience while working part-time as a clinical assistant, staff officer or associate specialist but the JCHMT does not recognise any of these as training posts.

The retainer scheme

The scheme exists to provide a toehold for doctors who are precluded from working for more than two sessions a week because of well founded personal reasons. The retained doctor is paid at the appropriate level for working sessions and undertakes to participate in a small number of continuing education activities in return for a modest honorarium. The emphasis is on retention in medicine, not training.

Note added in proof: The Department of Health has published a report on *Flexible training* (April 1993) which proposes ways of making part-time training easier to take up. The College has set up a working party on part-time training to investigate ways of implementing these proposals.

10 Management Training

General management exists and is thriving in the NHS. In many areas of the UK it has made little impact on clinical services, but in others the effect (both good and bad) has been dramatic. Consultants are under contract to provide health services under the NHS Acts in the district of their appointment. 'Who manages the service?' is the inevitable question. Although combined talents are necessary, a leader will need to have some general management skills to retain credibility.

The consultant's role

Within a district doctors can choose to perform their managerial role at one of three levels of expertise:

- As an interested (or non-interested) clinician with little or no managerial input
- As a clinician with a defined role within a department, ie taking the lead in representing the views of one's colleagues in the running of the department, or exercising a managerial role as clinical director
- As a clinician general manager with a leadership role across the service with all its resultant responsibilities.

Training requirements

Training in general management may be direct or indirect. Medical training offers an excellent indirect scheme for general management training. It provides the budding clinical manager with several invaluable attributes:

- A thought process that puts patients first
- Extensive general knowledge of clinical activities and in-depth experience within a specialty
- Scientific skills
- Ready access to a wealth of medical research, part of which is directly relevant to the provision of clinical services.

The major drawback of medical training is its narrowing effect on the doctor's perspective. The two major problems to be overcome by any doctor in management are: (a) the difficulties doctors have in dealing with populations rather than with individual patients; (b) the difficulties general managers have in dealing with individual patients instead of populations.

Direct skills in general management are gained principally by work experience and by attending courses at senior registrar level. A review of the management courses shows two main types:

- The beginners course which really has very little to do with general management but more with who does what, where and how in the whole NHS
- The intermediate course which gives an introduction to management skills, finance, personnel, communication, quality etc.

Everyone could benefit from a beginners course; those who wish to have a say in the running of their departments in the future should take the intermediate course. An alternative to the intermediate course would be to take some study leave to shadow a unit general and/or a district general manager, and see what they do from a distant and more objective standpoint.

Career prospects

There is as yet no department that offers senior registrars a management or business degree opportunity. This path may well be available within the next 5–10 years in selected centres.

11   How to Write an MD Thesis

There can be no hard and fast rules for the preparation of an MD thesis. Each university has different regulations and each thesis is unique. However, certain guidelines can direct the candidate on to the right track. The following tips are derived from our own experiences and from conversations with colleagues.

Before you start

Obtain the rules from the degree awarding university, because they vary in detail between universities. You can submit your thesis to the university from which you qualified or sometimes to the university in which you will have performed the research.

Next you must choose a project. The idea for it does not have to be your own, but you must have enthusiasm for it. Talk to as many people as possible about your idea. Write down very briefly (eg two sides of A4) exactly what you have in mind to do and ask for constructive criticism: better now than later. Ask: Is the idea a good one? Is it feasible? Will you be able to study what you want to, in the ways that you want? Most important, will it provide enough data for a thesis? The important people to ask are the advisers appointed by the university to which you plan to submit your thesis. They will help you answer these questions and explain the local rules.

The two principles of the research are that it should be original (ie has not previously been done) and that it must be your own work. The results do not have to be earth shattering or of major clinical importance, but the methods used must be scientifically validated.

Getting started

Once you have an idea for a project, do a thorough literature search to make sure that no one else has done the work before you. Take copies of important references because you will need them when you come to write the thesis, and make sure that the source reference appears on the photocopy. Arrange the references to previous research in chronological order.

Once you are satisfied that your project will provide enough original information, you can proceed. If you plan to do experiments or make observations on human subjects you will need to apply to the local research ethics committee for approval.

Observations

Start by asking a statistician for advice in designing the plan and to help you decide the size of the study; this includes the number of observations to make, and the number of subjects. If you have an idea what result to expect from your experiment the statistician can help you to decide how many observations you will need to get a significant result within prescribed confidence limits. This is called the power of the study.

Methodology

You need to know the details of the methodology you will use. You must learn the method and be familiar with all the problems and know how to deal with them as they arise. You will learn these as you go along. However, you should not start the project until you have mastered the method; otherwise your results will change as you progress up the 'learning curve'.

What are the errors in your method? You must be sure that the methods are well validated in the population you are studying. If they are not, then you must perform validation experiments. You need to know the inter-observer and intra-observer errors. What is the reproducibility of the method in the same subjects over given periods of time?

Analysis of data

Once you have collected your data, you will need to analyse them. Get advice from a statistician as to the most appropriate method. You may need to use a computer to help you with the analysis, but make sure that you understand what the computer is doing or you will not be able to interpret the results that it generates. Think of incisive ways of presenting your data as graphs or illustrations. Tables of results are boring to read. When presenting your data in the thesis it is important to present the actual results and not results derived from mathematical analysis. The examiner will want to look at the raw data, or at least some of them, to be sure that they are genuine and valid.

Flexibility

In most experiments something unexpected happens and will need to be explained. This often requires additional experiments to test the explanation. You should look critically at the results as they arrive. Do not wait until all of a series of experiments have been completed before looking at the results. You may find a fundamental flaw early on which you can correct without losing much time. You may find that your original idea was wrong but a new idea comes to you during the experiment. The best thesis is one that follows an observation with a logically planned series of experiments to test it.

Peer review

Try to find a local adviser to help you who should be experienced and approachable and someone whose judgement you trust. Show him/her your early results to assess the progress of your experiments and help guide you on the next step. He/she can be far more dispassionate and critical of your data than you can.

Writing the thesis

This is often said to be the worst part of doing an MD. Borrow several theses from the university library to see how they have been written and set out. Judge which ways of presentation appeal to you. Try to make it easy for yourself by doing as much writing as you can early on and continually throughout your research programme. For example, when you have completed your initial literature search, you can write the introduction. If your project comprises a series of separate experiments write each one up as a paper or presentation. This has many advantages. First, it makes you analyse your data as you go; second, it makes you put the experiment in context for the reader and makes you use the references you have collected; third, it submits your work to peer reviews which may expose flaws and give other ideas for further experiments; fourth, it stamps your name on the research subject so that if someone else is working on the same subject you have staked your claim; fifth, it provides you with a publication for your *curriculum vitae*.

The thesis will need to be typed and bound. You will write many versions before submitting the final copy, so a word processor is essential. Most university departments will have a word processor available for your use, but you may find it easier to buy one. The alternative is to pay a typist to type your thesis which will probably turn out to be as expensive in the long run.

Your thesis should not be too long. This is probably the commonest problem. Below is an outline of what you might include in each chapter.

Introduction

Review the previous literature but keep to the point. If it is not directly relevant to your work do not include it. Put the previous work into a historical perspective, so that the reader can appreciate the development of the field. Explain where your work fits into the whole, and how and why you decided to do it.

Methodology

Describe your methods in full and justify their use. Compare the methods you chose with others available and explain why you chose the ones you did. Detail the validation of your methods.

Experiments

The way you set out the rest of the thesis depends on the type of research you have undertaken. If the thesis comprises a series of experiments following in a logical progression, each experiment should have a chapter to itself with linking paragraphs at the end of each chapter leading on to the next. Summarise the conclusion at the end of each chapter and introduce the next. Raw data can be tabulated in an appendix at the end to avoid cluttering up the text. If the thesis comprises a single, large but multifaceted study, you will only need one chapter on methods. Try to report the different aspects of the results in separate chapters. Help the reader by summarising at the end of each chapter.

Discussion

You should write a chapter that brings together all the different parts of the research project. In that chapter you can put the results into a wider context by referring to the known literature in the field.

Abstract

It is necessary to write a short and punchy abstract of the whole research which usually goes at the front of the thesis. This is what most people will read, so take time over it and make sure it is as interesting as possible.

References

When you write the first draft of your thesis make sure that you write down in the text any reference you quote immediately you use it. If you do this you will not forget where you found the information that you are quoting. It is easier to quote references in the text using the authors' names and year of publication (eg Channer and Roberts 1988) to help remind you to which reference you are referring. List them in alphabetical rather than numerical order and then, if you forget one or find an important reference later, it is easy to add it to the text and your list; if you use numbered references, you will have to change all the numbers in the text if you forget one (or you can use 12a, 12b, 13 etc). Make sure that all the references are correct and that your list tallies with the text.

Illustrations

Where possible, illustrations should be the same size as the paper (usually A4) to avoid the unsightly bulging that occurs when photographs are stuck into the middle of a thesis. Photographs can be printed directly on to A4 paper suitable for inclusion in the bound copies. Provide legends for the tables and illustrations which make sense when read in isolation, and try to place figures and tables close to the text relating to them.

Proof-reading

Whoever types your thesis will make mistakes (even you). Be painstaking over proof-reading since even spelling mistakes need to be corrected before the thesis will be accepted by the examiners. It is often helpful to ask a friend or colleague to read the script as well — two pairs of eyes are better than one. Always check that the numbering of tables and illustrations corresponds to that in the text.

Submission

When you are satisfied with the final draft you will need to make several copies (depending on the individual university rules). Make sure to keep a copy for yourself. Then you will need to pay to have the copies hard-bound. Some universities insist on a *viva voce* examination after your thesis has been read by the examiners. This is usually to give the examiners an opportunity to discuss critical or ambiguous points in the thesis.

These guidelines are not intended to be exhaustive and we may have missed important points. However, the preparation of an MD thesis is a time-consuming and often exasperating experience. We hope that others may learn from our experiences and avoid some of the frustration we felt when things did not quite go according to plan.

Note added in proof
See Chapter 8, page 34

If the principles embodied in the Calman report[1] are adopted, they will change the method of training and accreditation. For example, the registrar and senior registrar grades would be merged and a more structured training programme introduced than the one currently in operation. Specialist training would be shortened overall, the number of trainee posts would be reduced and the GMC would award certificates for completion of training on the recommendation of the Colleges. These proposals would allow the EC directives to be implemented. A consequence of these changes will be a requirement for more consultants irrespective of other considerations requiring more consultants.

1. A report of the Working Group on Specialist Medical Training. *Hospital doctors: training for the future*. London: Department of Health, 1993.

PART 2

Individual specialties

Details of current guidelines for higher medical training in each specialty are given in the JCHMT Training Handbook. The latest edition can be obtained from the Training Office at the College.

General (internal) medicine

The consultant's job

A general physician may be defined as a consultant who is responsible for the care of unselected emergency medical referrals and who takes part in acute admission of GP-selected medical patients. Very few consultants are now appointed to purely general medical posts; almost all offer an associated specialty interest. However, the breadth of general medical experience in the pre- and post-MRCP years is clearly of great importance when a consultant appointment is being made, particularly in a district general hospital. In a teaching or regional referral centre many consultants do hold single specialty posts and, where a general medical component is included, this usually involves much less time during the week than the area of special interest. In a district hospital the number of sessions devoted to the area of specialist interest varies considerably between posts according to the particular needs of the area.

Training requirements

Since most senior registrar posts are associated with teaching hospitals or larger district general hospitals, senior registrar accreditation in general (internal) medicine is very unlikely to involve a purely general medical rotation. They gain experience by rotations through a number of specialty areas, in addition to taking responsibility for acute general medicine intake. The choice of enrolling for a particular specialty rotation is therefore determined by the senior registrar's own area of medical interest, chosen on the basis of experience gained during the senior house officer and registrar years. The choice also depends on the senior registrar's career intention of working in a specialist referral centre or district general hospital, since few district general hospitals employ physicians with only single specialty experience.

However, recent research and audit have indicated that in certain circumstances (eg asthma, diabetes, myocardial infarction) patients may fare better under specialist care than under the care of general physicians. But on unselected medical take, patients, particularly the elderly, do not always present with diseases of one organ system.

In a large teaching hospital it might be possible for single-organ specialists to see, for example, all diabetic comas, but this is not possible in most district hospitals.

What do GPs want from hospital consultants? In outpatients they want expert advice on specific problems of their patients and will choose the specialist clinic accordingly. However, when they send in patients for acute problems they expect the receiving physician to be knowledgeable in all branches of medicine and therefore they want the opposite—a physician in general (internal) medicine.

Career prospects

With the changes in career structure in medicine it is evident that a doctor will now have to decide on his or her particular area of interest much earlier—ie when at senior house officer level. Registrar posts, although still offering a major general medical component, will increasingly be linked to training schemes in a specialist area of medicine. It will therefore be important to bear in mind career prospects within that specialty when applying for a registrar post, as has been the case previously when considering a senior registrar post. Involvement in research work will be an important aspect of training for registrars and senior registrars in all training posts. Consequently, the opportunity for research in non-teaching hospitals will be improved, and this will continue into consultant posts.

The variety of conditions encountered in the general medical component of a consultant post is stimulating but requires continued postgraduate education after consultant appointment to keep fully up-to-date. Whilst work in specialist centres concentrates on a clearly defined area of medicine, general medical involvement requires a mind open to a wider range of medical conditions and complications. Therefore, despite the increasing pressure from the public to be seen by an expert within an appropriate specialist area, a general medical component of consultant work remains of great importance.

Paediatrics

Paediatrics has emerged as a major branch of medicine over the past 30 to 40 years and is an expanding specialty which offers a variety of satisfying and stimulating careers. Paediatricians are represented professionally both by the College, which holds overall responsibility for training, and by the British Paediatric Association which was founded in 1928 to further the study of child health and promote friendship among paediatricians. A large number of paediatric specialties is now available to the trainee. Details of these training programmes are included in the JCHMT's blue book. For the majority, experience in the corresponding adult specialty is not actually necessary (although some trainees may arrange to have this experience for research or other reasons). Experience in the relevant paediatric specialty is essential.

The consultant's job

Paediatricians are likely to remain among the busiest physicians in terms of hours of work and call-out rates. They also need to be able to work as part of a team with their colleagues in child psychiatry, teaching, the nursing professions, speech therapy, physiotherapy, social work and so on. Most of all, paediatricians must be able to communicate with parents in order to achieve optimal health for their child patients.

Training requirements

The post-registration period of general professional training at SHO level should include wide experience of acute general paediatrics and neonatal medicine, together with experience in paediatric specialties, paediatric surgery and community child health. Many will wish to add breadth to their training by taking posts in related disciplines such as general medicine, obstetrics and general practice before sitting the MRCP examination.

At registrar level, there are many excellent posts involving rotation between paediatric specialties and experience in both teaching and district general hospital units. Trainees will also be able to develop research interests at this stage, and many will proceed to a period of full-time research towards an MD or PhD. Those planning a career in a certain paediatric specialty will also need registrar experience in the equivalent adult specialty in order to obtain dual accreditation. The accreditation requirements for community paediatrics demand experience both in hospital and in community child health.

At the time of publication, the move from registrar to senior registrar is probably the greatest hurdle for the aspiring paediatrician. Most senior registrar posts offer the intending general paediatrician opportunities to continue research and to develop a special interest.

Career prospects

Although the number of paediatric consultant posts has recently been increased, many have remained unfilled owing to a shortage of adequately trained senior registrars. This applies especially to posts that provide neonatal intensive care in district maternity units. Community child health is also an expanding specialty and follows the recommendation of the Court Report that consultants should be responsible for preventive paediatrics and the care of children outside hospital. So far, there have been about 100 such consultant appointments in England and Wales, and a further 200 posts are planned, with a corresponding increase in senior registrar numbers.

Because of the present dearth of appropriate senior registrar rotations in community paediatrics, a number of senior clinical medical officer posts are being approved for training on an individual basis.

Academic medicine

The term 'academic medicine' in this context indicates that the trainee will pursue a career in which, at every stage, medical research will be a major component. Careers of this type vary greatly in their content, ranging from those who do full-time research straight after registration and never go back to clinical practice, through those who try to combine clinical practice and research as part of a post in a clinical academic department, to NHS consultants who opt to have one or two research sessions. Similarly, the type of research varies widely and ranges from basic scientific work through more conventional patient-orientated clinical investigation to clinical epidemiology and health service research.

The consultant's job

The majority of clinically trained academic clinicians form part of university academic departments. They usually divide their time between a limited amount of clinical practice, research and teaching. Because of the central role of academic departments in teaching centres, increasing seniority brings a good deal of administrative work both in the university and in the NHS.

Training requirements

The training of academic clinicians varies enormously depending on their future aims. A few individuals who wish to make a career in full-time research go straight into a research post after their preregistration jobs and usually obtain a PhD at this stage. They then work in various post-doctoral positions doing full-time research and do not return to clinical practice. Those who are contemplating this type of career should probably move straight into research after their house-jobs because if they find that they are not suited to this type of career they can always move back into standard clinical training after they have completed their first three years of research.

However, most clinical academics would continue to complete their general professional training after their house jobs and take the

MRCP diploma. They would then break off for a minimum of three years to do full-time research, obtaining, if they so wish, a higher degree such as a PhD or MD. The critical step is to find a place in a well organised laboratory or research centre where a proper training in research methods is available. This normally would take a minimum of three years and perhaps a year or two longer. Funding for this period can be obtained through MRC or Wellcome Trust training fellowships or other fellowships of this type given by the medical charities. Afterwards, they can return to clinical medicine and complete their training for accreditation. They would then aim to obtain a lecturer or senior lecturer post which will give them time to organise their lives between a limited amount of clinical practice and research. This type of career pathway is suitable for those who wish to do more basic science or clinically orientated research.

This type of training programme would be appropriate for those who want to move up the ladder in university academic departments. It is also possible to continue full-time research after such a programme and not return to clinical practice. However, to obtain an honorary consultant contract as a member of the clinical academic staff, a period of accredited training in a specialty is normally required.

Career prospects

Most British clinical academic departments are quite small and usually have one or at the most two professors, with a reader and one or two senior lecturers. Because of the large administrative load carried by senior academics, anyone who wants to sustain a good level of research throughout their career is best advised to try to 'stick' at the senior lecturer/reader level or aim for a personal chair. The prospects for those who plan to make a full-time career in research are somewhat limited. A few academic clinical departments are able to take on individuals of this type. Posts may be obtained in MRC institutes or units, and the large cancer charities also have such career posts. The Wellcome Trust's senior fellowships are a good entrée to this type of career and the Trust is now creating a few career posts at the principal fellowship level for particularly gifted individuals. It is also possible to have an academic research career in a preclinical department, although here too the number of posts is very limited. Some may be tempted to go abroad but career research posts are not easy to come by, and even in the USA those who are doing almost full-time research in academic clinical departments would be expected to have some clinical training along American lines. Anyone who wants to pursue this direction is advised to go to the USA as soon as possible after registration because British higher qualifications are not recognised there.

Accident and emergency (A & E) medicine

This specialty is almost 20 years old and still developing. The majority of consultants are full-time and come from a variety of backgrounds. Most of the full-time consultants in post hold the FRCS, but a significant proportion hold the MRCP. The early growth of the specialty was limited by the number of suitably trained applicants but this is no longer the case. Competition for posts is keen and it is anticipated that the increase in the number of consultants will continue to grow for the foreseeable future. The British Association for Accident & Emergency Medicine is the professional body which represents and co-ordinates the specialty, and the Emergency Medicine Research Society provides a forum for the discussion of research topics.

Plans by the Royal Colleges of Anaesthetists, Physicians and Surgeons to form an intercollegiate faculty are well advanced.

The consultant's job

An A & E consultant is responsible for all the patients who present to the A & E department. Resuscitation of the acutely ill and injured takes priority and is the particular *forte* of this specialty. Management of cardiac arrest and the multiple injury patient are the two areas in which the A & E doctor has a great deal to contribute. Most A & E consultants develop a special interest, often based on their backgrounds, eg hand surgery if surgically trained, or poisonings if medically trained. There is a small number of paediatrically trained A & E consultants who work in paediatric A & E departments. A feature of A & E medicine is that the working day is usually unstructured and the variety is enormous. 'All human life is here' and one can move from sophisticated resuscitation for a severe cardiac problem to the treatment of alcoholism or a child with a cut knee. The requirements are a broad background in both medical and surgical disciplines and the ability to keep cool in a crisis. Casualty departments are informal, and relationships between various specialists and disciplines are undefined. It is essential to be able to co-operate with nursing and ambulance staff on an equal level.

Many A & E consultants become involved in out-of-hospital rescue work and the higher training of ambulance crews. Disaster management and planning is an increasingly important part of the work of an accident and emergency consultant.

Training requirements

Most A & E departments are staffed by senior house officers, sometimes in inadequate numbers. The Department of Health (DoH) considers registrar posts in A & E orthopaedics as posts in A & E. These are orthopaedic training posts; there are only a handful of pure A & E registrar posts. The specialty is negotiating with the DoH to rectify this anomaly and an expansion of the registrar grade is planned. This will eventually allow entry to the specialty at registrar level. For the foreseeable future, a consultant will be the first in line on call after the SHO in many departments. What this entails in terms of emergency call-out depends upon what other facilities and local arrangements are available at the hospital concerned.

Entry for training in A & E medicine is at present at senior registrar level, and there are about 65 posts available, but soon enrolment at career registrar level may be possible. No further expansion of the senior registrar grade is planned for the immediate future. Candidates must have the FFA, FRCS or MRCP(UK) and a broad-based background. Accreditation will require a period of at least five years from enrolment with the JCHMT, of which at least two must be as SR. The training programme is tailored to ensure that areas not covered by previous experience are made up. Most senior registrars therefore spend some time in paediatrics and intensive care as well as in psychiatry and general practice. If their training has been predominantly medical, they spend at least three months in general and orthopaedic surgery, and if predominantly surgical, in medical and psychiatric posts. It is now possible to take the second part of the FRCS Edinburgh in A & E medicine and surgery. Candidates are eligible to sit this examination if they have been qualified for four years, have Part 1 of the Membership, or the primary Fellowship or the primary FFA of any of the Colleges, and have completed 12 months A & E, 12 months acute general medicine and 12 months general surgery. Senior registrars may spend some time abroad during their training and the JCHMT will recognise appropriate experience.

Career prospects

Accident and emergency medicine is expanding and is now an established specialty. In the past it was thought that A & E departments should be staffed by one physician and one surgeon; now the feeling is that they should be staffed by two specialists in A & E medicine. Career prospects are good.

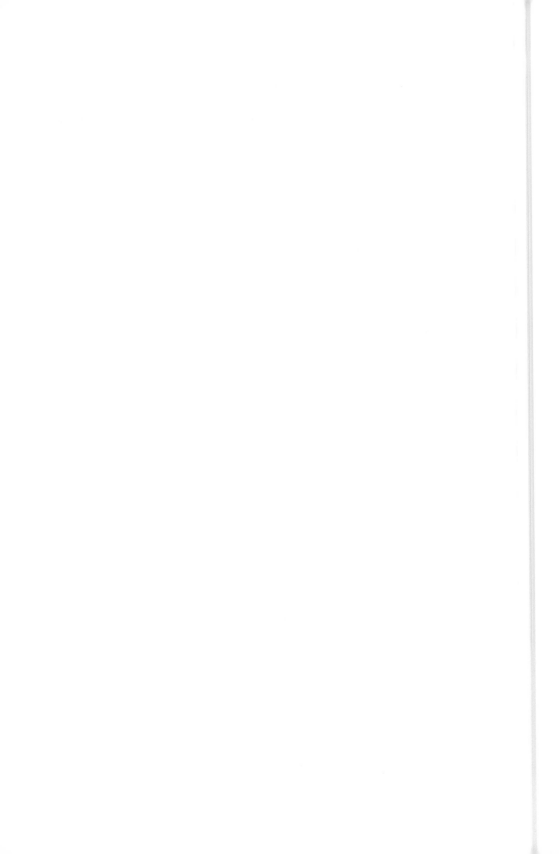

Cardiovascular medicine

Major changes in the practice of cardiology in the past decade have necessitated changes in both the training of senior registrars and the types of cardiology consultant post available.

Cardiology has always been a highly competitive specialty. It is even more attractive nowadays because of the advances in diagnostic techniques and the opportunities to intervene effectively in cardiac disease with powerful new drugs, interventions and surgery. It is very rewarding for the 'hands on' physician.

The consultant's job

With the provision of Doppler echocardiography and the refinement of nuclear cardiographic techniques combined with exercise stress testing, the physician with an interest in cardiology can assess patients with cardiac disease in the district general hospital and make decisions about the need for surgical intervention in valvular and ischaemic heart disease. Hence, more patients can be assessed locally, thereby reducing the referral rate to the regional cardiac centre. In the light of these technological advances, which are within the budget of the district general hospital, there has been an increase in the number of posts for physicians with an interest in cardiology. This increase has been fuelled by pressure from the British Cardiac Society and the Royal College of Physicians Cardiology Committee, whose biennial survey highlighted regional differences in the provision of cardiology services. More recently, aggressive early management of acute myocardial infarction with intravenous thrombolytics has also demonstrated the need for cardiological expertise in every district general hospital. It is likely that there will be a steady increase in the number of posts for cardiologists to satisfy this unmet need. Most cardiologists based in DGHs will also have some responsibility for general medicine.

Within the regional cardiac centres, cardiologists provide an invasive service. Patients referred for surgery usually require coronary angiography. Permanent cardiac pacing is also usually a regional or subregional service. Technological advances have changed the practice of cardiology here also. Angioplasty and valvuloplasty have spawned a new breed of interventional cardiologist. Technical advances in pacing and the further understanding of cardiac electrophysiology, especially with the development of surgery for arrhythmias, have necessitated specialist cardiac electrophysiologists. Hence, within a modern regional cardiac centre there may be cardiologists with specialist skills and interests.

Training requirements

After completing general professional training it is usually necessary to begin to learn cardiological techniques at registrar level in a regional centre. Appointment to senior registrar grade requires some expertise in pacing, cardiac catheterisation and echocardiography. Research experience is also necessary and many senior registrars will have obtained a higher degree during their time as registrar, often by spending 1–2 years in a research post.

The training programme for physicians in cardiovascular medicine has changed recently to take account of this, and higher specialist training can now begin at registrar level. Of the six years of training, five should be spent in cardiology with at least two in active clinical work at registrar and two at senior registrar level, including two years in a centre with cardiac surgery. The specialist training should include clinical experience in general cardiology and some paediatric cardiology. Improvements in surgical techniques have allowed more children with complex congenital heart disease to survive into adult life; exposure of the trainee to the diagnosis, management and problems of these patients is important. Technical expertise in cardiac catheterisation and angiography, cardiac pacing, echocardiography, exercise stress testing, ambulatory monitoring, nuclear cardiography and acute coronary care remain an important part of training, much of which can only be provided by time spent in the regional cardiac centre. Trainees should also have some knowledge of strategies for the prevention of cardiac disease and rehabilitation of patients after myocardial infarction and surgery.

One year of higher specialist training is spent in general medicine. The final year of training allows the trainee to develop a specialist interest. This gives the trainee the opportunity to design training to suit a particular type of cardiology post. For example, emphasis on the non-invasive assessment of cardiac disease would be important for the physician with an interest based in a district general hospital. The College recommends a further two years training for interventional cardiologists in order to provide adequate 'hands on' experience. The JCHMT also insists that the training programme includes adequate opportunity for research, a regular teaching commitment and medical audit.

Paediatric cardiology

The original subspecialist cardiology posts were in paediatric cardiology. These posts are few and are limited to regional or supraregional paediatric cardiological centres. Most trainees who enter the specialty have a background of general paediatrics although some physicians enter from adult cardiology. Currently there is a shortage of adequately trained senior registrars to fill vacant consultant posts but this is likely to be short-term and it is unlikely that senior registrar numbers will be increased. Paediatric cardiology, like adult cardiology, has changed dramatically in the last decade and now diagnosis is often entirely echocardiographic. Again the opportunities for intervention using catheter techniques are developing; for this reason trainees still require the skills to catheterise often very small babies. It remains a very challenging and rewarding specialty but physicians have to be able to work within a team since surgery is fundamental to management in many cases.

Career prospects

Currently the numbers of senior registrars training and consultant posts available in cardiology are well matched and it is intended to match registrar numbers with senior registrar numbers. This has been achieved by careful audit of the specialty over the last decade by the British Cardiac Society and the Royal College of Physicians Cardiology Committee. It is predicted that by the late 1990s there will be more consultant posts available than senior registrars in training. The prospects look good, but there remains a major bottleneck at senior registrar level where there are two or three registrar posts for every senior registrar post. Eventually the bottleneck will be at SHO level.

Clinical genetics

Clinical genetics is a new and expanding specialty but some regions at present do not have adequate clinical genetic services. Clinical geneticists should ideally be based in a regional genetic centre where there are appropriate supporting staff and associated genetic laboratory services. Genetic clinics are held in the regional centres and in satellite clinics in association with local clinicians.

The consultant's job

Genetic conditions can affect all age groups and all body systems, so a broad clinical background is essential. Day-to-day work is varied and includes diagnosis of genetic conditions, genetic counselling, ward referrals, acting as an information source on genetic matters for colleagues, liaison with genetic laboratories and clinical colleagues in investigations and clinical interpretation of results, and in prenatal diagnosis of fetal defects. More recently, clinical geneticists have been involved in clinical application of recombinant DNA technology and in research in this exciting field. Teaching of undergraduates, post-graduates and associated professional groups is an important aspect of their work. Most clinical geneticists are not in charge of hospital beds but can admit patients by arrangement with consultant colleagues.

Entry to the specialty is usually at senior registrar (SR) level although entry at registrar level may become increasingly common in the future. There are thirteen NHS-funded senior registrar posts in the UK and a number of *ad hominem* SR equivalent posts funded by limited-duration research money. Before entering the specialty the trainee should have post-registration general professional training, ideally to include both paediatrics and general medicine, leading to the MRCP. An SHO job in obstetrics has been seen as an advantage by some. A year may have been spent in the study of basic genetics, either as a postgraduate or during undergraduate training in the form of an intercalated BSc. Senior registrars without this basic genetic qualification will be seconded to learn basic genetics during higher specialist training. As senior registrar, a trainee should gain knowledge of dysmorphology, biochemical and population genetics, cytogenetics,

DNA technology, the genetics of disorders of different body systems and genetic counselling techniques. Encouragement is given for research projects leading to an MD degree.

Career prospects

It is recommended that there should be one consultant clinical geneticist per million population. Though this target is far from being achieved, the NHS appears to be moving towards it. If these hopes are realised, career prospects should be good if regions expand to recommended levels. Trainees for other specialties may wish to acquire training in genetics, and dual accreditation may be possible in some cases. The Clinical Genetics Society, which consists of physicians, scientists and other professional groups working in the field, meets twice yearly and encourages contributions and attendance by younger members.

Clinical immunology

The compass of clinical immunology is determined by pathogenetic mechanisms of disease, regardless of tissue site. This is conceptually attractive, offers considerable potential in therapeutic terms and is particularly useful in the management of multisystem diseases, but requires up-to-date understanding of many of the organ-based specialties. However, much of the work is typically carried out in conjunction with other specialists. Clinical immunology also has a strong laboratory component, bridging clinical medicine and pathology. In many settings, immunopathology was the first aspect of the specialty to emerge, offering a range of diagnostic laboratory tests for immunologically mediated disease with a consultative role largely based around this service.

During recent years, developments in medical practice have underlined the need for 'physician immunologists' with a primarily clinical axis. These developments have included: an increasing appreciation of the prevalence of allergic diseases; the emergence of AIDS; the widespread use of therapeutic immunosuppression; the extension of transplantation to more organ systems; the increasing characterisation of lymphoproliferative disease; and an expanding appreciation of the importance of autoimmunity in multisystem disease.

The commonest immunologically mediated disorders are allergic diseases. While most allergic disorders can be managed in general practice and medical specialties, specialist evaluation and treatment of severely affected cases is essential. Paediatric immunology is based on a few referral centres, supported by paediatric subspecialties.

The consultant's job

The role and working relationships of physicians in clinical immunology will vary according to the local prevalence of immunologically mediated diseases, the existence of other clinicians with expertise in such disorders and the extent of immunopathology provision. Whether or not there is an immunopathologist, the physician immunologist or organ-based specialist with an interest in immunology will have a significant role in the diagnostic immunology services and in clinical liaison. A physician immunologist or a designated organ-based specialist with an interest in immunology may take direct responsibility for patient care for some disorders and will provide a clinical consultation service for patients referred by general practitioners and hospital consultant colleagues. The balance will vary among the various immunologically mediated diseases.

As well as underpinning the need for a firm immunopathology diagnostic base in clinical centres, there is a need for physicians with immunological expertise and training to provide either direct clinical care or consultation services.

Training requirements

A new training programme has been drawn up for physician immunologists, and training programmes in organ-based disciplines have increasingly incorporated immunological aspects. New training posts in clinical immunology at senior registrar level have been approved, with further posts to follow as consultant expansion occurs.

Experience is required in relevant clinical medical specialties and in laboratory aspects of diagnostic immunology. Substantive training posts in clinical immunology and immunopathology are ideal for those pursuing a primary career as physician immunologists. In addition, there are a number of full-time or part-time postgraduate courses in immunology; research posts in clinical or laboratory work are also of considerable benefit to the trainee.

Career prospects

While there are relatively few specialist immunology posts, many other medical disciplines require immunology training and expertise, and in some cases organ-based specialists with such expertise can act to provide a clinical immunology service. It is often wise for the trainee to ensure accreditation in another discipline so that it is possible to achieve consultant status as physician immunologist or as an organ-based specialist with additional expertise in immunology.

Clinical pharmacology

Clinical pharmacology is one of the more recently recognised specialties in medicine, but it has previously existed in one guise or another (materia medica, therapeutics). It is not 'organ based', has no clear service commitment to offer and, at present, flourishes largely within an academic environment. These factors may have hampered its development. Clinical pharmacologists in training were rarely considered for appointment to consultant posts, as they could not offer any special service to a clearly defined group of patients. Many retrained in another specialty and have been appointed as physicians with an interest in diabetes, cardiology or geriatrics; some have found a niche in acute poisoning. While there has been some expansion of clinical pharmacology posts in medical schools, there are a mere handful of posts in the NHS. The British Pharmacological Society provides the principal forum for presentation of scientific research and professional advancement of the specialty.

The consultant's job

Clinical pharmacologists should be physicians first and foremost. In addition, they should help develop rational drug prescribing policies within their hospitals or health authorities and be the catalysts for research projects and clinical trials. Some may take on special responsibility for certain disorders, eg hypertension, epilepsy or acute poisoning; others may also provide a service to other physicians and general practitioners on difficult therapeutic problems such as drug adverse effects, drug interactions, and the rationalisation of complicated regimens. A drug information service is now increasingly provided by hospital pharmacists.

Training requirements

After training in general medicine at SHO and registrar level, the aspirant should obtain a senior registrar post in general medicine with clinical pharmacology in a recognised unit. These days it is probably wise to select a particular organ or system for intensive study, as this increases the options when applying for consultant posts. During the senior registrar appointment a knowledge of methods of investigation of drug action in man should be acquired in addition to pharmaco-kinetics, clinical trial methodology, statistics and the clinical management of acute poisoning. Most are best learned by doing one's own clinical trial(s) or research project(s). Clinical pharmacologists must be good communicators, so it is important to acquire high standards of lecturing ability, research presentation and scientific writing. An MD or PhD is an essential qualification which is obtained during the senior registrar appointment, but the trend is towards completing the project while in a research post at registrar level.

Career prospects

The present problem is that many a young doctor finds the subject appealing and is attracted to the idea of becoming a consultant clinical pharmacologist. Academic units need good, enthusiastic, young doctors who will teach and also undertake research. There is no shortage of excellent applicants for research or lecturer posts in clinical pharmacology. But after a suitable time in such posts the goal of becoming a consultant clinical pharmacologist is often not realised. Many have then entered the pharmaceutical industry—a decision very few regret.

Despite the poor prospects, there are many avenues for those who are clinical pharmacologists at heart. Very few senior registrar posts exist for those who are committed to clinical pharmacology alone. Many senior registrar posts in general medicine with another specialty as a primary interest have a period attached to a clinical pharmacology unit. This is perhaps the best approach, for there are serious doubts about the value of an accreditation certificate in clinical pharmacology alone. Other posts offer triple accreditation, ie general medicine, clinical pharmacology and one other (cardiology, gastroenterology or endocrinology). From these it is possible to apply for consultant jobs in the specialty other than clinical pharmacology. Once appointed consultant the interest in clinical pharmacology may be developed. For those who set their sights on an academic career there may be slightly better prospects, but the present incumbents of chairs of clinical pharmacology look remarkably youthful.

Communicable and tropical diseases

Infections and their consequences are essentially preventable, yet they consume an enormous amount of health care resources and they remain important causes of morbidity, disability and premature death. For these reasons they currently have a high public profile and there is increasing pressure on health service managers and medical staff to limit the human and financial consequences of infectious disease. Consultants in communicable and tropical diseases, working in one of the most clinically and scientifically rewarding areas of modern medicine, play an essential role in this process.

The consultant's job

For physicians specialising in infectious disease, community acquired infections still provide a major part of the work-load. Some physicians care predominantly for adults, others for both adults and children. Because the specialty is not organ based, competence as a general physician and/or paediatrician is essential.

In district general hospitals, clinical infection teams, in which the infection physician works in close partnership with medical microbiologists, are becoming increasingly important. As a member of the team the clinician will be expected to assess patients thought to pose a cross-infection hazard, and to advise on the management of bacteraemia, PUO, imported infections, and infections in intensive care situations and in compromised hosts. Antibiotic management will be an integral part of this consultation process.

An increasing number of individuals with HIV infection or AIDS present to clinical infections services. The infection physician caring for such patients will often take lead responsibility in a multidisciplinary team and will work closely with other AIDS specialists and agencies.

Parenteral drug use has become a major problem in many urban centres, and drug users provide a challenging array of infections for diagnosis and management.

Imported infections often threaten life but expertise in this area is thinly spread. Infection physicians therefore play a crucial role in the early detection and management of these diseases. Some clinical units maintain high security facilities for viral haemorrhagic fevers, eg Lassa fever.

The other important responsibilities of the infection specialist include advice and assistance with infection control, immunisation and travel medicine, and collaboration with other consultants in control of communicable disease and in hospital control of infection teams. Some consultants have formal sessional commitments to public health medicine.

Training requirements

Guidelines for training in the specialty have recently been published by a joint working party of the Royal College of Physicians and the Royal College of Pathologists.

After completion of general professional training, and after the MRCP(UK) has been obtained, all trainee physicians must gain experience in certain core disciplines; arrangements for the remainder of their training should be variable and flexible.

a *Core disciplines*
  i Sound experience in general (internal) medicine is essential.
 ii Trainees must work for at least one year (at senior registrar level) in an infectious diseases unit in a teaching hospital or approved regional centre.
iii Such courses as the DTM&H or the MSc in clinical tropical medicine provide valuable training in tropical and imported infections. Alternatively expertise may be gained in suitable centres overseas.
 iv Trainees would benefit from experience at the bench in a micro-biology laboratory for at least six months to understand the meaning, potential and limitations of laboratory investigations.

b *Options for further training*
  i Additional clinical experience in general medicine or paediatrics (preferably with experience in oncology or transplantation).
 ii Further training in medical microbiology or parasitology (eg MSc, DipBact).
iii Training in basic epidemiology.
 iv Research in a laboratory discipline related to infectious diseases, perhaps leading to an MD or PhD. Suitable disciplines include molecular biology and studies of the host response to infection.
  v Training in medical microbiology, virology or immunology leading to the MRCPath.

Career prospects

Manpower statistics for the specialty indicate the need for substantial expansion in the number of consultants. The Royal College of Physicians and the Royal College of Pathologists are currently pressing for the number of consultant posts in England and Wales to be increased.

The discipline of clinical infection is understandably very popular among young clinicians, and the challenge is now to provide the outlets needed for their enthusiasm at career level. A significant expansion of clinical infection services would release much accumulated expertise, with immediate benefits in patient care.

Dermatology

Dermatology is an enjoyable and stimulating specialty dealing with patients of all ages presenting with a wide variety of disorders. It includes not only purely dermatological problems but also many systemic diseases. Recent therapeutic advances have greatly improved the management of some of the more severe forms of common dermatoses such as psoriasis and acne. Greater interest in surgical techniques has increased the dermatologist's involvement in the management of malignant melanoma and other skin cancers.

The consultant's job

Most consultant dermatologists work in more than one health district. The majority of the work is on an outpatient basis. Diagnostic biopsies and the treatment of skin tumours form part of everyday practice. Inpatient beds may be centralised to provide for several districts and dermatologists or may be shared with the general physicians within a district. In teaching hospital departments there are dermatology trainees at senior registrar and registrar grades with senior house officers in a minority of departments. In district general hospitals a house physician or senior house officer is often shared with one of the medical teams. Additional medical staff in the outpatient clinics is provided by clinical assistant posts. It is becoming increasingly common for district general hospital departments to employ staff grade doctors and overseas visiting registrars. Dermatological disorders are the commonest reason for time lost from work. As a result dermatologists are frequently asked to provide reports for industrial compensation claims or for legal cases brought before the civil courts claiming damages.

Training requirements

MRCP and three years post-registration general professional training are required before entering dermatology at registrar level. A minimum of four years clinical experience in dermatology, at least two at senior registrar level, is currently recommended for accreditation in the specialty. The majority of registrar and senior registrar posts are at teaching hospitals but may involve time in district general hospitals either as part of a rotation or as clinical sessions. There is provision for part-time training as a registrar as well as on the supernumerary senior registrar part-time training scheme which is advertised annually by the Department of Health. Training includes experience in dermatological surgery, histopathology of the skin, mycology, patch tests and phototherapy. The diversity within the specialty allows interests from the psychological to the surgical to be pursued. Research is encouraged. Some time spent purely on research can be allowed for accreditation. Similarly time spent abroad working in dermatology may be counted for accreditation but it is important to check beforehand that the proposed work and venue are appropriate.

Career prospects

There has been an increase in the number of trainees in recent years and the number of accredited senior registrars exceeds the number of consultant posts potentially available over the next few years. Most trainees will therefore spend more than the recommended four years in training. This should not deter those planning to enter the specialty as the same situation applies to most branches of medicine. In addition, there will be many changes in the NHS in the next few years and no one can predict how this will affect career prospects.

Diabetes and endocrinology

In the UK there are general physicians with a special interest in diabetes. There are also posts with more emphasis on pure endocrinology and those which combine diabetes and endocrinology.

The consultant's job

The majority of physicians with an interest in diabetes and endocrinology work in district general hospitals, sharing on-call commitments with other general physicians. A consultant might expect to spend 40% of his or her time on general medicine, 40–50% on diabetic services and 10–20% on endocrine diseases. The majority of endocrine cases will have thyroid disease, the remaining 20% covering the range of glandular disorders and also reproductive problems.

In smaller district general hospitals one consultant is likely to deal with all endocrine and diabetic problems. The consultant will usually work with an SHO or a registrar or possibly both. A clinical assistant is likely to help in the diabetic clinic. Diabetic services extend beyond hospital boundaries to include shared care with general practitioners and community care mediated by diabetes specialist nurses. Close liaison with other specialists such as ophthalmologists, nephrologists, obstetricians, orthopaedic and vascular surgeons is necessary for successful patient management.

There are only about 50 pure endocrinologists in the whole of the UK, mainly in the larger referral centres and working closely with neurosurgeons, radiotherapists, oncologists, paediatricians and gynaecologists. Most have a senior registrar or a registrar, plus an SHO, sometimes with additional research staff. Several large academic units specialise in endocrinology and offer good opportunities in basic and clinical research.

Training requirements

Training requirements for specialising in diabetes and endocrinology can perhaps be deduced from the experience of the hundred or so consultants newly appointed in this field over the past five years. The median age of appointment was 37 years. Successful candidates had obtained a good grounding in medicine by spending about three years in general professional training whilst obtaining their MRCP. Just over four years were spent at registrar grade, half in clinical work and half in research. Some held a PhD; most had an MD, having completed the work for a thesis or even having written it up by their time of appointment to the senior registrar grade. Diabetes and endocrinology lend themselves well to both basic and clinical research. About two years in the laboratory is certainly worthwhile and provides a realistic understanding of hormonal and other assays.

Career prospects

The selection pressure upon potential physicians is changing. Until now, the promotional bottleneck has been between registrar and senior registrar grades, most senior registrars becoming consultants sooner or later. JPAC proposals will now reduce the number of senior registrars and registrars in training in England and Wales to balance predicted consultant requirements. This will move the bottleneck to the interface between the SHO and registrar grades over the next ten years. Even so, the practice of diabetes and endocrinology is enjoyable so the specialty is likely to remain popular.

Gastroenterology

In the UK there are an increasing number of hospitals where two consultants share the gastroenterological and general medical workload.

The consultant's job

The majority of gastroenterologists in the UK are appointed as general physicians with special experience and training in gastroenterology. It continues to be a popular career choice, perhaps reflecting the opportunities for involvement in diagnostic and therapeutic techniques as well as providing general patient care. A commitment to general medicine, including rotas for acute medical admissions, is usually expected although there is a growing demand for an increasing proportion of the consultant's time to be spent on diagnostic and therapeutic endoscopy. Specialist centres for hepatology and gastrointestinal physiology have been established and physicians totally devoted to gastroenterology are on the increase.

The newly appointed gastroenterologist should be proficient in diagnostic and therapeutic endoscopy. The work may involve supervision of enteral and parenteral feeding and the management of acute and chronic liver disease, including bleeding oesophageal varices. Joint management by physicians and surgeons is increasingly practised and provides optimal standards of care for certain disorders such as inflammatory bowel disease and gastrointestinal bleeding.

Training requirements

The trainee will spend three years as an SHO in specialties which need not include gastroenterology. Clinical training at this time should provide a balance between service commitments and an educational programme in order to secure Parts 1 and 2 of the MRCP. Traditionally, a registrar post with an interest in gastroenterology would then be obtained, ideally spending one year in a teaching centre and one year in a district general hospital.

The introduction of *Achieving a balance* will however modify this career structure. Research leading to either an MD or PhD thesis is highly desirable and may in future be carried out before obtaining a career registrar post. Some research posts will be available for career registrars. If during or after such a research period the individual changes career direction, the experience obtained will remain advantageous in pursuing a chosen career. Two or three years will be spent as registrar and a further two or more years at senior registrar level will complete higher medical and gastroenterology training.

Career prospects

The backlog of senior registrars awaiting promotion has been virtually cleared and in future the major obstacle is likely to be the career registrar post. Having achieved such a post, promotion to consultant grade should be anticipated. During the next few years, demand for consultant gastroenterologists will outstrip supply of senior registrars who may expect consultant status after three years in post.

Genito-urinary medicine

The specialty of genito-urinary (GU) medicine in the UK is long established, well organised and respected worldwide. Departments of genito-urinary medicine see 670,000 new patients annually, a threefold rise in 15 years. There are about 230 clinics, most of them in the precincts of district general or teaching hospitals. The consultants in the specialty are supported by clinical assistants, doctors in the training grades, nursing staff and health advisers—contact tracers.

The consultant's job

Patients present with a wide variety of clinical conditions and also personal, social and psychiatric problems. However, many of the conditions are curable, an unusual situation relative to many other medical specialties, and this results in a high degree of job satisfaction. GU medicine is largely an outpatient specialty but most departments have access to inpatient facilities as well as close links with many other hospital departments. Most patients attend direct without first seeking advice from their own doctor. Departments of GU medicine play a pivotal role in the prevention and management of HIV infection. This includes the provision of counselling and health education to those at risk as well as the challenging management of the broad spectrum of disease manifestations.

The problems of HIV infection and of infection with hepatitis viruses, human papilloma viruses and herpes viruses attract many physicians into GU medicine who might have pursued a career in mainstream infectious disease or general medicine. Although perceived largely as an outpatient specialty, many GU physicians play an active role in the management of inpatients.

In addition to undergraduate and postgraduate teaching duties, doctors in this specialty are responsible for health education of young people. Requests for help in this respect from various organisations are increasing.

Training requirements

To enter the specialty a higher diploma is necessary, either the MRCP or MRCOG. Those with the MRCP must have had clinical experience in gynaecology and those with the MRCOG in general medicine. During the four years of higher medical training, experience of dermatology and microbiology is desirable. The large numbers of patients attending clinics and the close links with microbiological departments provide excellent scope for clinical, epidemiological and microbiological research.

Annual courses in sexually transmitted diseases are held in Liverpool and twice yearly in London. The Medical Society for the Study of Venereal Disease meets six times a year when lectures and original scientific papers are presented. The society publishes its own journal— *Genitourinary Medicine*, formerly the *British Journal of Venereal Diseases*.

Career prospects

GU medicine is a growth specialty and the current prospects for doctors who have trained appropriately are excellent. The good prospects and the different but satisfying work pattern with largely young people have attracted many well qualified doctors to full- or part-time consultancies in the specialty. Few regret their choice of career.

Geriatric medicine

An enthusiastic but realistic approach to the investigation and management of old people presenting with a variety of symptoms is the *raison d'être* of geriatrics, which still is a truly general specialty. Doctors make positive choices to enter the specialty. Research and teaching in geriatric medicine continue to expand. Integration of geriatric and general medical acute services is taking place in many hospitals, partly as a result of the need to reduce junior doctors' working hours.

The consultant's job

Besides acute general medical care, geriatricians are involved in rehabilitation of old people as well as in some aspects of long-term care; hence the necessity to work as part of a multidisciplinary team. The population base is changing and geriatric medicine is rapidly evolving. There are opportunities to be involved in the planning of new and exciting services in hospitals and the community.

Geriatric medicine covers a range of facilities often on multiple sites which combine local accessibility with central specialist services. This enables the provision of a seamless service. Junior staff may be trained in all aspects of hospital, day hospital and domiciliary care.

Training requirements

Initially wide general medical experience is needed and MRCP is essential. Time spent in related fields such as general practice, neurology or psychiatry will prove to be useful. A short time spent working in a geriatric department is recommended before committing oneself to specialty training. At present this occurs at senior registrar level, although this may change as the role of career registrar posts in geriatrics becomes clearer.

Although it is possible to opt for single specialty accreditation, or dual accreditation in geriatrics and general medicine, care should be taken when opting for single accreditation since this may significantly limit the choice of a consultant post. Recruitment to the specialty is improving and, although clinical experience and commitment remain most important, it is increasingly necessary to develop research skills and a special interest backed with publications. Academic geriatrics is also expanding.

Career prospects

Geriatric services range in type from one totally integrated with general medicine to one based remote from the district general hospital. The majority of posts are wholly in geriatric medicine, but an increasing number are combined posts as 'consultant physician with special responsibility for the elderly'.

The consultant opportunities for senior registrars thus look more encouraging than in most other medical specialties. Opportunities for part-time training exist in this specialty and women are well represented.

Haematology

Haematology is an exciting and expanding branch of medicine that offers the unique combination of clinical responsibility for patients with management of a diagnostic laboratory service.

The consultant's job

Patients of all ages are treated as both in- and out-patients. The spectrum of disease is wide, encompassing the malignancies, bone marrow failure and immunosuppression, haemorrhagic and pro-thrombotic states and the more common anaemias. It calls for wide clinical experience including familiarity with intensive care support, reverse barrier nursing, techniques of prenatal diagnosis and counselling skills. Haematological complications of pregnancy, systemic disease and associated treatments ensure close liaison with most specialties. In addition, haematologists have responsibility for the laboratory services of the hospital and district. This includes routine diagnosis, blood transfusion and coagulation as well as the more specialised tests for haemoglobinopathies, enzyme and vitamin assays, immunopheno-typing and molecular biological techniques. As head of the department the consultant has managerial responsibilities for quality assurance, organisation and training of staff, budget management and forward planning.

Training requirements

Training requirements reflect this diversity. MRCP and three years post-registration general medical training are usually required before entering haematology at registrar level. Junior staff are usually shared with the consultant general physicians. MRCPath Part 1 (two written papers) may be taken after three years of haematology experience. MRCP no longer gives exemption. MRCPath Part 2 (an oral and practical examination lasting three days) is taken after five years of full-time approved training, at least two years of which must be in a post recognised for higher specialist training. Research experience is increasingly important and best achieved during registrar and senior registrar posts.

Career prospects

As with several other specialties, the number of trained haematologists being produced exceeds the number of consultant vacancies annually available. Traditionally, haematology has been a popular specialty for women (23% of the consultant posts). However, in any single-handed post more than a full-time commitment is required.

Intensive care

This is a young specialty which began in the late 1950s and initially only dealt with patients who had respiratory failure, but now includes acute medical disasters, multiple trauma and post-operative care after cardiothoracic surgery, organ transplantation and neurosurgery. Since that time the ability to support other organ systems has increased. It is now commonplace to support the cardiovascular system, kidneys, liver and provide artificial nutrition. Intensive care of patients requires facilities for mechanical ventilation, acute peritoneal or haemodialysis, haemofiltration, temporary cardiac pacing and invasive haemodynamic monitoring. Continuous monitoring of the ECG, vascular pressures, EEG or intracranial pressure may be necessary in some patients. If an intensive care doctor is to make a real contribution to patient care, training must have been received in these techniques. The institution and management of such therapy therefore requires a firm grounding in clinical medicine with a special emphasis on cardiovascular and renal physiology and pathology.

The consultant's job

By its very nature, intensive care medicine is a costly specialty both in terms of staff and equipment. The type of patient referred often depends on facilities provided by other specialties in a particular hospital. A survey by the College of 168 intensive care units found anaesthetists in administrative charge, while patient care remained with the admitting team or was shared with an anaesthetist in nine out of ten admissions. With the change in emphasis away from pure respiratory care to multi-organ support, more physicians are becoming actively involved in the care of critically ill patients; some have executive responsibility for the intensive care unit as well as clinical responsibility.

Training requirements

At the present time there is no clear training structure for this specialty in Britain but plans are well advanced to establish an intercollegiate committee of the Royal Colleges of Anaesthetists, Physicians and Surgeons to oversee the development of a diploma in intensive therapy. There are specific intensive care training posts for physicians at both the SHO and senior registrar grade (although these latter posts are open to senior registrars of other specialties as well). Trainees must spend at least one year in a post approved for general (internal) medicine after completing their GPT. Necessary technical skills may be acquired during training in anaesthesia (airway management in particular) as well as in posts in chest medicine, cardiology or nephrology. A further period working abroad in Australia, America or Scandinavia is encouraged.

Career prospects

The personality of a doctor working in intensive care is important since the job will involve contact with most colleagues in the hospital and the establishment of good working relationships will be essential. The consultant in intensive care must be able to lead a large team of doctors and nurses. Although intensive care medicine can be very satisfying when a moribund patient is restored to health, the mortality for many conditions that require such care remains high. The intensive care physician must accept that a high proportion of patients will not survive.

Medical oncology

The young doctor who wishes to develop a hospital career which will involve the management of patients with cancer currently has two choices, medical oncology or radiation oncology (radiotherapy). The term 'clinical oncologist' is confusing and should be abandoned. Seventy percent of the medical oncology posts are based in university departments, provided by research fund endowments, whilst most radiation oncology posts are NHS funded.

An increasing trend in recent years has been the creation of integrated cancer treatment centres, generally based in teaching hospitals, where medical oncologists and radiation oncologists work together. This system has met with widespread approval and provides increasing opportunities for common training and joint patient management. However, the roles of the medical oncologist and radiation oncologist remain distinct. While both are heavily involved in care of patients with all types of cancer, the medical oncologist should be chiefly concerned with systemic forms of treatment, particularly in patients with cancers which are sensitive to chemotherapy, eg lymphomas, testicular cancer, breast cancer, small cell lung cancer and ovarian cancer. In addition they should take the leading role in the evaluation of new agents for patients with the less responsive forms of cancer. The radiation oncologists will be principally involved in radiation therapy and will share the responsibility for the management of patients with many common forms of cancer. In centres where no medical oncologist is present, the radiation oncologist will also have a major involvement in the use of chemotherapy.

Medical oncology is an increasingly research-based specialty and many medical oncologists, especially those in university departments, will devote part of their time to participation in laboratory and/or clinical research projects. On the other hand, there is a limited number of individuals in district general hospitals who combine general medicine with a special interest in medical oncology. Close collaboration between these individuals and cancer treatment centres is necessary, and this pattern of care has proved successful in ensuring optimal management of cancer patients in hospitals which may be some distance from cancer treatment centres.

Training requirements

The JCHMT guidelines for training in medical oncology stipulate a minimum training period of seven years following the completion of preregistration training.

It is essential that medical oncologists have a sound training in general medicine and this should be acquired through at least two years of SHO/registrar posts in general medicine. A third year at this stage, giving additional experience in a relevant area, is recommended.

Higher medical training will be pursued in a post accredited for training in medical oncology alone or for medical oncology and general medicine. All aspects of cancer should be included. The trainee should become familiar with a wide range of management problems and the psychological and social needs of cancer patients. Detailed knowledge of the use of systemic therapy and experience in new treatment evaluation should also be acquired.

During this time it is desirable to spend approximately two to three years in original research. This may involve molecular or cell biology, pharmacology, immunology or other relevant topics. Requirements for accreditation are flexible, and many trainees will spend time on a laboratory project before entering higher medical training. In any event, those seeking accreditation in medical oncology must have spent a minimum of two years in clinical senior registrar posts approved for higher medical training in medical oncology.

At present there is no postgraduate examination in medical oncology. It is conceivable that the first stages of higher medical training in medical oncology will be integrated to some extent with those in radiation oncology.

Career prospects

Medical oncology in the UK is a young specialty, with a history of less than 30 years. Projections for the future are uncertain, but over the past five years new consultant posts in medical oncology have been created at the rate of two or three per year, mostly in cancer treatment centres. A continued gradual expansion of this type of post as well as of the 'physician with interest' is envisaged as new more demanding treatments become available.

Metabolic medicine

This is a broad-based specialty in which physicians who have been trained in different clinical specialties and basic science methods may gain accreditation. Physicians in metabolic medicine will usually have trained in general internal medicine and care of patients with metabolic disorders of acquired or inherited origin. However, they may have interests in inherited diseases, clinical molecular biology, clinical genetics, disorders of calcium and phosphate homeostasis, acid-base balance, electrolyte disturbances, lipid disorders and the metabolic response to stress or clinical nutrition. A training in basic sciences at some stage in the career of the physician is essential. There are very few posts at present in metabolic medicine, but this specialty is likely to expand as the demand for the application of the recent advances in molecular genetics for the management of clinical disorders is likely to increase. In addition, the future goals of gene therapy will also require appropriately trained physicians. Individuals trained in metabolic medicine are more likely to be employed in research and teaching centres.

The consultant's job

A consultant in metabolic medicine would be expected to spend a maximum of 40% of the time in clinical medicine and 60% pursuing research. Junior staff will usually be an SHO or registrar or both on the clinical side with much of the work centred in the outpatient clinic or day-care wards. In addition, there will be work with basic scientists and responsibilities for training PhD students and clinical research fellows. Close liaison with other specialists such as diabetologists, endocrinologists, obstetricians, clinical geneticists, chemical pathologists, nephrologists, radiologists, immunologists and paediatricians is necessary for successful patient management.

Training requirements

During general professional training some relevant experience may be gained in a post which has special interest in metabolic disorders or

91

in related fields, eg diabetes, endocrinology, nephrology or intensive care. In addition, three to four years training in basic science research, eg molecular biology, is desirable; this may be combined with higher specialist training during which time experience in general (internal) medicine and metabolic disorders is gained. This period should be directed towards gaining an MD or PhD (or both), as these are desirable for further progress. An intercalated science qualification (BSc or BA) at undergraduate level is helpful. The essential feature is that the training should lead to a wide understanding of the metabolic origins of disease and of appropriate clinical investigation and management. Knowledge of the principles of genetics and molecular biology is highly desirable.

Career prospects

This specialty is likely to expand as the demands for the application and understanding of molecular genetics and gene therapy increase. In addition, the investigation and management of patients with metabolic disease integrates the principles of the preclinical specialties, ie biochemistry, physiology and pharmacology, with the clinical specialties. Thus, the practice of metabolic medicine is rewarding and enjoyable and is likely to become more popular. The selection pressures upon physicians in training are changing. Previously the career prospects between registrar and senior registrar were limited, with the majority of senior registrars eventually becoming consultants. With the reduction in the numbers of senior registrars and registrars in training to achieve a balance with the predicted consultant requirements, the career limitation has now occurred between the SHO and registrar grades. These features are also true of most other medical specialties. However, because recruitment to the specialty of metabolic medicine is from such a broad and diverse field, it is difficult to define a precise path to complete training for a consultant grade. The emphasis in this specialty is to enable physicians to gain substantial training in clinical and basic science methods so that British academic medicine can continue to flourish.

Neurology and clinical neurophysiology

Neurology is a small specialty which has always been highly popular and competitive. The training structure and prospects have remained fairly stable and predictable, and it has been spared the severe manpower problems of many specialties. Consultants work at 40 neurological/ neurosurgical centres in the United Kingdom and every health region has at least one.

The consultant's job

Neurology appeals to people who enjoy 'bedside' diagnostic medicine and patient contact; basic clinical skills remain of paramount importance. Neurology consists mainly of outpatient work, and the majority of patients are managed without recourse to specialised investigations. However, there have been enormous technological advances in the last decade and neurologists now need to be conversant with a wide range of investigative techniques. It is undesirable for neurologists to work in isolation and the majority of posts are based in teaching hospitals with sessions on one or two days a week in district general hospitals within the region. There is an increasing trend for neurologists to have a primary district general hospital role, working, for example, six sessions in the district but having four sessions a week at the teaching hospital centre. Many district general hospitals now have their own CT scanners which makes the neurologist more independent of the teaching hospital. Brain MRI scanning is increasingly available but at present confined to the teaching hospitals which will also provide neuroradiology, neurophysiology, neuropathology and neuropsychology, together with inpatient facilities for neurology and neurosurgery. Liaison with ophthalmology, ENT and, of course, general medicine is close.

Junior staff in training are largely based at such centres where a group of four to six consultants might have, for instance, one senior registrar, two registrars and two SHOs. Preregistration posts are unusual in neurology. In some areas facilities are not centralised and a single neurologist may be based at one large hospital and have some specialist facilities elsewhere. The vast majority of neurologists do not subspecialise, though, since neurology encompasses such a wide spectrum of disease and with the growing application of basic medical science, there is ample scope for special interests.

Training requirements

General professional training may include one year in clinical neurology, neurosurgery, psychiatry, or research in related basic science subjects. Higher professional training is spent in an approved neurological centre with an additional recommended year in psychiatry, neurosurgery, applied neurophysiology or basic neurological science. The usual course is to spend three to five years as a medical SHO and registrar while obtaining the MRCP, then, as an entrée into a specialist centre, many aspiring neurologists become a neurology SHO before going on to be a neurology registrar, the latter for approximately two years.

Career prospects

Competition is fierce throughout, particularly for senior registrar posts. However, the number of senior registrar and consultant posts is fairly well matched, so that obtaining a senior registrar appointment almost guarantees a consultant post. In order to be appointed to a senior registrar post it is almost essential to have an MD (or equivalent thesis degree), and this means at least two years of full-time research, usually after a neurology registrar appointment. Thus, it is unusual to become a consultant neurologist less than 10–12 years after registration. The importance of keeping early career options open by making the general professional phase of training as broad-based as possible cannot be overemphasised. Alternative career avenues beyond the stage of neurology registrar are very limited.

Clinical neurophysiology

Clinical neurophysiology is a smaller but expanding specialty with a shortage of adequately trained applicants to fill senior registrar and consultant posts. The development and clinical application of such techniques as evoked potential studies, ambulatory EEG, video recording and specialised muscle recording methods are resulting in expansion of the number of consultant posts. Newly appointed consultants have a varied training which usually includes periods in general medicine, paediatric, clinical neurology, and as a senior registrar in clinical neurophysiology; they usually possess the MRCP and a higher research degree, eg MD in a basic science. Senior registrar posts are limited to large regional neuroscience units.

Nuclear medicine

Nuclear medicine is a branch of clinical medicine, the distinctive feature of which is the use of radioactive material. It embraces all applications of radioactive materials in diagnosis or treatment or in medical research, with the exception of the use of sealed radiation sources in radiotherapy. The techniques of nuclear medicine are now well established and should be available to all patients.

The physician wishing to become a consultant in nuclear medicine should have some special interest in basic science including basic physics, instrumentation, radiochemistry, radiopharmacy, and radiation dosimetry and protection.

The consultant's job

At present nuclear medicine services are provided by consultants in nuclear medicine, by radiologists with special interests in nuclear medicine, by physicians with special interests in nuclear medicine and occasionally by radiotherapists. One of the demanding aspects of the subject is its diversity. The nuclear medicine consultant's advice may be sought on a complex renal problem, then on a cardiological, an oncological, a surgical or an endocrine problem, all in the space of a few hours.

A nuclear medicine physician may wish to specialise in particular areas. For example, one might choose research on bone diseases and the use of radioactive tracers in their diagnosis and follow-up whilst another may be attracted to cardiological work. The central responsibility will be to provide a general diagnostic and therapeutic service.

Training requirements

The training recommended by the Intercollegiate Standing Committee includes four years in a post approved for higher training in a department of nuclear medicine for a person who wants to be a consultant in nuclear medicine, one year of specialist training in an approved post for a person who will be a radiologist with an interest in nuclear medicine and two years specialist training in an approved post for a person who will be a physician with an interest in nuclear medicine. Before starting this training they should hold MRCP, FRCS or an equivalent qualification.

Nuclear medicine has now been accepted by the European Community as a monospecialty and it is envisaged that more consultant posts should be created. Furthermore, it is possible that one-third of the consultants presently in post will retire within the next ten years, thus requiring the increased number of training posts.

Occupational medicine

Occupational medicine is a relatively new and expanding specialty which is concerned with the effect of work on health, and of health on work, and has a major preventive as well as treatment role. There is now extensive legislation relating to health and safety at work and this has encouraged the wider provision of occupational health and safety services.

Professional representation is through the Society of Occupational Medicine which currently has more than 2,000 members, of whom about 900 work full-time. The Faculty of Occupational Medicine was established in 1978 and now has 1,700 Fellows, Members and Associates.

The consultant's job

The primary role is to advise workers, management and trade unions on all health matters with the aim of preventing ill-health and promoting good health. This is a clinical and preventive discipline which requires a detailed knowledge of occupational diseases and expertise in health assessment, rehabilitation, toxicology, environmental assessment and control, the application of epidemiological and statistical techniques, and much enthusiasm. As industries evolve, new processes may create new hazards and perhaps new occupational diseases, so there is always a challenge. Issues such as stress, alcohol, drugs and AIDS are growing in importance, as is occupational mental health which requires good behavioural and psychological skills. Boredom is rarely experienced.

The problems of different industries—eg aviation, chemical, mining, steel, National Health Service, retail—lead to much subspecialisation. As well as the experience described, the occupational physician also needs to acquire managerial and communication skills, as one day he or she may have to justify the departmental budget to the tough financial scrutiny of industrial line management, and on another speak at a mass meeting of workers concerned about an unfamiliar hazard and then justify the recommendations made. The specialty is unusual in that most posts are outside the NHS, though this is an expanding area with consultants being appointed in many districts.

Facilities vary, depending on the nature of the industry, but normally include provision for the treatment of illness and injury at work, for critical health evaluation and often physiotherapy or rehabilitation services.

A trained occupational physician will be experienced in industrial chest radiology, pulmonary function assessment, audiometry, toxicology, skin and allergy testing, and many will develop other skills.

While large industries have well established occupational health services, the majority of physicians may work alone or with perhaps one colleague and a team of occupational health nurses and part-time GPs. The effective provision of occupational health care involves teamwork with other related disciplines such as occupational hygienists, nurses and safety practitioners. Epidemiology and research are fundamental to the role: identification of an occupation-related health hazard often involves assessment of the health of the group as well as of the individual.

Training requirements

Entry to the specialty is normally after the completion of general professional training, and the MRCP(UK), though desirable, is not mandatory; currently 82 training posts are approved. GP training and experience is valuable and many occupational physicians enter the specialty through general practice. Attendance at an academic course is possible on a full-time, day or block release, or distance-learning basis, and is strongly recommended. Associateship of the Faculty is gained by examination, and Membership is awarded after satisfactory completion of training and the acceptance of written work. The age distribution within the Faculty is skewed towards the older range, so there will be many job opportunities. The occupational physician has many career options, and there is considerable mobility. Occupational physicians with wide experience are in demand. Few occupational physicians should expect to work for a lifetime in one organisation.

Palliative medicine

Palliative medicine is primarily involved with the care of patients with malignant disease but is also concerned with care for patients with diseases such as motor neurone disease and AIDS. Doctors who wish to work in palliative medicine will require a sound training in general medicine and a broad understanding of the treatment of primary and secondary malignant disease including medical, surgical and radio-therapeutic approaches to treatment. In addition, an appreciation of the roles of non-medical staff in the care and support of the patient and family and knowledge of the possibilities and limitations of care in the community is essential. It is also necessary to understand the management of psychological problems faced by patients and their families and of the process of bereavement.

The consultant's job

The consultant in palliative medicine will provide the highest possible standard of medical care for patients in or outside the hospital, with particular emphasis on the rapid and effective control of pain and other distressing symptoms. He or she will recognise the emotional, social and spiritual needs of patients and families and seek to deal with them as part of a multidisciplinary team. The consultant will work in close collaboration with hospital and community based services, regularly reviewing medical procedures and drug therapy and keeping abreast of research developments intended to improve patient care. Teaching is an integral part of the consultant's role and consultants are increasingly involved in health service management.

Training requirements

Those intending to practise with a full-time commitment in palliative medicine will normally undertake four years of higher specialist training, including two years in specialist units that offer a full range of services in different settings, eg inpatient care, outpatient clinics, home care, bereavement services. An elective period of research or special experience of some aspect of palliative medicine is desirable.

Not less than one year, and up to two years, may be spent in general medicine and other relevant specialties, eg oncology, infectious diseases, radiotherapy, haematology, geriatric medicine or approved general practice. Those intending to practise in a specialty other than palliative medicine/terminal care would gain similar experience over a period of one year in a specialist unit dealing with end-stage malignant disease.

Career prospects

Career prospects in palliative medicine are good. So far, there are not many candidates for appointment at consultant level, as few have spent time in the existing senior registrar posts. Doctors with good relevant experience in other specialties but without the extensive experience of palliative medicine now regarded as mandatory may still be successful at consultant appointments committees. At the present time various higher qualifications are acceptable for those entering specialist training in this new specialty but there is now much competition for the approved senior registrar posts.

Pharmaceutical medicine

Pharmaceutical medicine is a discipline concerned with the discovery, development, evaluation and monitoring of medicines and the medical aspects of marketing. Like public health medicine it deals with populations of patients and individuals, but draws heavily on medical skills achieved through general medical training.

Physicians have historically been an important part of the process of introducing new therapies in medicine. Originally called medical advisers, physicians have been employed in pharmaceutical companies for much of this century and the first professional support group, now called the British Association of Pharmaceutical Physicians, came into being in 1957. The Dunlop Committee, which was formed in 1963 to formalise the regulation of registration and marketing of therapeutic substances, reinforced the need for physicians in industry and in government.

The increasing responsibilities of the discipline, which became known as pharmaceutical medicine, include legal accountability under the Medicines Act for drugs in research, the regulatory submissions and monitoring of risk/benefit of drugs once they are on the market. Such responsibilities require special skills and in 1975 the Royal College of Physicians initiated a diploma in pharmaceutical medicine to encourage training in the discipline, and in 1989 the Faculty of Pharmaceutical Medicine was inaugurated.

Jobs in pharmaceutical medicine

Careers in pharmaceutical medicine encompass three main groups of physicians: those working in the pharmaceutical industry, those with appointments within regulatory bodies such as the Medicines Control Agency (MCA) and those working in independent research organisations dedicated to the development of new medicines. As very few of the jobs in the discipline conform to a conventional medical structure there is no clear-cut point where a fully trained pharmaceutical physician becomes a consultant. Similarly there is a wide range of jobs with different levels of responsibilities ranging from the director of the MCA and industry divisional heads with hundreds or even thousands of staff through to medical directors in specialist areas with one or two assistants. The jobs with greater responsibilities require not only training in basic pharmaceutical medicine but many years of experience and dedication. Such pharmaceutical physicians also need to acquire highly developed skills in financial and other aspects of management.

There are several subdisciplines in pharmaceutical medicine which include:

- research and development—working on drugs before they are on the market;
- phase IV—working on drugs which are on the market;
- drug surveillance physicians—dealing with adverse events of drugs both in research and on the market;
- regulatory physicians—working on submissions either for the regulatory agencies or in the agencies themselves.

One pharmaceutical physician may be responsible, with his or her team, for all the clinical development of one or more compounds. The development programme must effectively evaluate the risk/benefit which can be a major challenge in a discipline which is by definition always working on the frontiers of science.

It is essential that good communication is maintained across the world so that effective and efficient drug development can be conducted and adverse event surveillance can be maintained within companies and regulatory authorities.

Training

Entrants into the discipline should have undergone a period of general professional training. Many will have higher medical degrees (though not necessarily MRCP), PhDs or MDs. Perhaps because the discipline has many research based jobs it also attracts people with an intercalated BSc. During the first two years the new entrant is expected to gain a substantial knowledge base which will build upon basic medical training. Subjects such as toxicology, pharmacology, clinical pharmacology and clinical trial and programme design are expected to be understood to a greater depth. New subjects are also required, such as a detailed knowledge of regulatory requirements throughout Europe and in the US, the concept of planning and management of large research and development programmes, the legal, ethical and other aspects of information, promotion and education about medicines and the economics of health care.

New entrants should have spent two years in pharmaceutical

medicine before presenting themselves for examination for the Diploma in Pharmaceutical Medicine which will enable them to obtain Associateship of the Faculty of Pharmaceutical Medicine. During this period they are strongly advised to seek counselling from a Faculty supervisor and also to undertake some formal training which is available in different courses.

Membership of the Faculty of Pharmaceutical Medicine will be obtained by completion of a dissertation and an oral examination usually after a further two years in jobs within the subject. During this period entrants will be expected to demonstrate from their dissertation that they have gained the many skills such as project management, writing and presentation and teamwork in addition to detailed knowledge of a particular subdiscipline.

Career prospects

Many pharmaceutical physicians trained in the UK now live in North America or in European countries (currently estimated at over 20%) illustrating the truly international nature of the discipline. There are many exciting career opportunities within the subject; most carry a great deal of sometimes exhilarating responsibility which may not be readily apparent. Most are as part of other large organisations (pharmaceutical companies or government departments) and are just as subject to organisational politics and structural hierarchies as the NHS or academia.

Public health medicine

Public health medicine is concerned with the promotion of health and the prevention of disease within whole communities. It has a key role in assessing the health needs of communities, in advising health authorities on the formulation of their district procurement plans, in the setting of contracts with provider units, and in the monitoring and evaluation of service delivery through these contracts.

Every health authority has a department of public health medicine headed by a director of public health medicine (or chief administrative medical officer in Wales and Scotland), with one or more other consultant colleagues, and in many districts one or more doctors in the training grades. Public health physicians also work in regional health authorities, special health authorities, government health departments, Medical Research Council units, universities, and the armed forces.

Public health medicine complements clinical medicine, which concerns the health of individuals, by focusing on the health of populations. Epidemiology is the science fundamental to the practice of public health medicine, and the skills which must be acquired are population control of communicable and non-communicable diseases, statistics, computing, health economics, nutrition, social and public policy, organisational theory, behavioural science, health education, communication and management.

Training requirements

Training for a career in public health medicine has many similarities to that for other specialties but there are some important differences. First, because the basic sciences of the specialty have such a small place in undergraduate teaching, it is necessary to provide a special academic input. Currently this is undertaken either full-time for one year by attending a Master of Science course at selected universities, or part-time for a longer period by attending courses arranged by various consortia of university departments of public health medicine. This situation is about to change, however, with the establishment by university departments of a number of schools of public health medicine which will provide locally based one-year courses leading to a Master of Public Health degree.

Second, service training in public health medicine provides experience in a number of topics which relate to clinical medicine but do not feature to any great extent in junior hospital posts or general practice vocational training. Examples would be epidemiological studies, health needs assessments, planning and evaluation of services, infectious disease control, health education and health promotion. This affects the timing of the specialist qualification, the examination for the Membership of the Faculty of Public Health Medicine. The MFPHM Part 1 tests the candidate's knowledge and understanding of the basic sciences and should be completed before entry to higher specialist training. The MFPHM Part 2 tests the candidate's ability to apply these basic skills to public health medicine problems and is usually completed during the tenure of a senior registrar post.

Third, in public health medicine a single training grade covers both registrar and senior registrar posts. This means that, once appointed, the doctor usually stays within the same region for the five years of training. In some instances this will involve a formal rotation round two or more different district health authorities within the region, whereas in other instances the doctor holds an appointment at a single district for the five years but has the opportunity to arrange short-term attachments to other units.

Public health medicine attracts applicants from a wide variety of medical backgrounds, with a minimum of two to three years post-registration experience in clinical posts including training for general practice. For those entrants to the specialty with considerable clinical experience, either in hospital or in general practice, special arrangements can sometimes apply, with reference both to shortening the length of the training programme and to the provision of protection of salary.

Those wishing to consider a career in public health medicine are encouraged to obtain a copy of the booklet *Public health medicine: training, examination regulations and syllabus* from the Faculty of Public Health Medicine, Royal College of Physicians, and to meet the Faculty adviser for their region, whose name can be obtained from the Faculty of Public Health Medicine.

Career prospects

Career prospects are good because of the effects of the retirement of a cohort of older doctors, and a current expansion in the number of consultant posts to meet the challenges set for the recently re-orientated specialty. In 1989 there were 100 vacant consultant posts in public health medicine in the UK. There were approximately 360 doctors in training posts and many new training posts being created to parallel the expansion in consultant posts. Prospects for the future are bright. The success rate for eventually obtaining a consultant post in the NHS, having been accepted as a trainee, is in the order of 75%, which compares very favourably with many clinical specialties.

Rehabilitation medicine

The lack of specialist care for adults with disabilities is a notable defect of today's health service. In 1972 the Tonbridge report recommended that there should be a consultant in rehabilitation medicine in every district. In November 1989 the Department of Health formally recognised rehabilitation medicine as an independent specialty in England and Wales, though it has been well established in Scotland for some fifteen years.

The consultant's job

The consultant practising in rehabilitation medicine will have to work closely with colleagues of all disciplines as well as with the many other professionals in health and social services. Useful qualities to possess are clear thinking, good communication skills, the ability to work as a member of a team, unlimited patience and political and managerial skills. The constant fight for extra resources and facilities for disabled people is a time-consuming but important part of the job.

Rehabilitation medicine is a broad specialty which can encompass some specialist areas, such as amputee rehabilitation and rehabilitation after spinal injury. At a district or community level, priorities for this specialty are young disabled people in the transition from school to adult life, those with multiple disabilities, including cognitive impairment (such as those with traumatic brain injury), those requiring special training or support in order to remain in their own home or at work, and requiring specialised equipment particularly in relation to orthosis, special seating, environmental control equipment and specialised wheelchairs. It is envisaged that most consultants will practise exclusively in rehabilitation medicine (RM). A small minority will probably have sessions in other specialties related to rehabilitation medicine such as neurology or rheumatology, but specialists with dual qualifications will be expected to spend at least six sessions a week in rehabilitation medicine. Those involved in more specialist areas will normally be full-time in the specialty.

Training requirements

Rehabilitation medicine is one of the more expedient specialties for those who wish to pursue part-time training. Apart from the need for basic training in general medicine, experience in other specialties such as neurology, rheumatology, psychiatry, mental handicap and geriatric medicine is an advantage.

There can be few areas of medicine where there is such scope for research of direct and practical relevance to patient care. The full potential of new materials and technology has yet to be realised in the treatment of disabled people and there are many established rehabilitation techniques which would benefit from scientific evaluation. The Society for Research in Rehabilitation is the foremost academic society in rehabilitation in Europe. It is an interdisciplinary society which holds regular meetings at which such work can be presented. The British Society for Rehabilitation Medicine is open to medical graduates of all grades and specialties interested in the field of rehabilitation medicine. It holds scientific meetings as well as representing the political interests of those training and practising in the field.

Career prospects

There is a growing appreciation of the need for new training posts in this field and at the time of writing it is proving difficult to fill all the consultant posts that are being advertised.

The number of senior registrar posts approved for full-time training in RM was increased in 1990 to 25 in England and Wales. A further 15 posts are currently approved for joint training in rehabilitation medicine and rheumatology, but in future the balance is likely to shift strongly in favour of full-time RM posts.

Renal medicine

The relatively low incidence of renal disease within the adult population as a whole means that extensive clinical experience in this specialty is denied to physicians in other disciplines. Renal disorders often complicate multisystem diseases and careful management may avoid or delay the necessity for expensive renal replacement therapy. The investigation and management of primary and secondary renal disease encompasses all areas of general medicine, and an extensive and comprehensive clinical background is important. There is often an overlap with the management and investigation of patients with hypertension and metabolic disorders, broadening the scope of the specialty. Dialysis and transplantation are expensive resources, and consequently are often centralised at a regional site, usually within a teaching hospital, but sometimes supported by satellite dialysis units elsewhere in the same region. Renal medicine is very much an 'acute' specialty, and junior staff are often much busier than their contemporaries in other areas of medicine. The nature of the specialty and its specialisation ensures a broad base for clinical and scientific research.

The consultant's job

Within a large regional unit the consultant usually works as one of a team of consultants, often with responsibility for a particular clinical area of expertise, such as transplantation or dialysis. There is close integration with other disciplines, including diagnostic radiology, nuclear medicine, immunology and urology. Much of the consultant's work is outpatient based, and because of the regional nature of the specialty this may often involve satellite clinics at other hospitals. Supervision of the day to day running of a large renal unit in terms of acute admissions, hospital referrals and the routine investigation of patients is often on a rotational basis with consultant colleagues. This allows 'reservoirs' of time to pursue specialist clinical interests or research. The renal unit relies on a cohesive structure with highly trained nursing and technical support staff. Renal replacement therapy is an expensive resource and requires the development of administrative skills on the part of the clinician, and indeed became one of the earliest targets for the application of resource type management.

Consultants appointed to posts outside regional units sometimes also hold honorary clinical contracts at their regional centre. These posts may often include a commitment to acute general medicine in a district general hospital setting and perhaps the supervision of a satellite dialysis unit. Junior staff in this environment are often less experienced and 'thinner on the ground', so the practical skills of the consultant may still be called upon. Single-handed appointments of this type are often arduous in terms of the workload involved, and arrangements for specialist cover for annual and study leave may be difficult.

Training requirements

Competition for senior registrar posts in renal medicine, which are usually dually accredited for higher professional training with general (internal) medicine, is high. This necessitates intensive training at a general level in specialties which should include exposure to intensive care and acute general medicine. A period of clinical or laboratory based research is essential as most candidates competing for senior registrar posts usually have completed work toward or have written their MD or PhD theses. Such research is usually timed to follow a period of training at registrar level so that a specific area of clinical or scientific interest can be identified. The objectives and financial support for a research project should be well defined at the outset and clinical duties should only encroach on such a project to the bare minimum.

Career prospects

Currently there are only just over 100 consultant posts in renal medicine in the United Kingdom. Vacation of these posts or creation of new posts is at a rate of approximately four to six per year. Direct comparison with other European countries suggests that the provision for renal services in the United Kingdom is very much below demand, and there is considerable pressure to expand staffing at consultant level by at least 100%. In order to manage the growth rate in terms of referral of patients with renal disease, some of this expansion may well be covered by the provision of tenured posts at a staff grade level.

Respiratory medicine

Respiratory medicine is undergoing a period of change at present, both in work practices and staffing patterns. There has been a rapid expansion in thoracic investigative and therapeutic techniques to include diagnostic procedures using the fibreoptic bronchoscope for transbronchial biopsy and for laser therapy for tumours. Improved imaging techniques with high resolution CT scanning and NMR imaging, and also physiological and immunological assessment of respiratory disease, make diagnosis a more precise process. The respiratory physician no longer deals solely with tuberculosis or chronic bronchitis but with a much wider spectrum of disease which includes autoimmune lung disease, asthma, occupational lung disease, adult cystic fibrosis, lung cancer and the management of pulmonary infections in the immunocompromised patient. With the sequencing of the cystic fibrosis gene, and probably in the next few years the atopy gene, it is likely that gene therapy will be part of the treatment regimen for these diseases in the foreseeable future.

The consultant's job

About three quarters of respiratory consultant posts are also responsible for general medical patients and take part in the acute unselected 'take'. These physicians usually work in district general hospitals. The respiratory monospecialist usually works at a referral centre, often in a teaching hospital, and has less involvement with general medicine.

Training requirements

Training for respiratory medicine is at present in a state of flux because of the proposed merger of the senior registrar and registrar grades and the organisation of career registrar rotations. At present no such rotations exist in respiratory diseases, but appropriate training programmes are now being organised. It is likely that on entry to the registrar grade there will be two years of training in respiratory medicine and general (internal) medicine which may be recognised for HMT and which would include experience in chest radiology, including

scanning and bronchography, fibreoptic bronchoscopy and allied
techniques, respiratory intensive care and also other diagnostic and
therapeutic skills. This may be followed by a two-year research period
in a specialist thoracic medicine department and then by two years of
higher professional training at senior registrar level in general and
respiratory medicine before applying for accreditation and/or a consultant post. Budding academic doctors would probably obtain a
lecturer post or an MRC training fellowship following or during the
registrar period to further their research experience. In future it is
hoped to provide a degree of flexibility during higher professional
training so that the incumbent could take a sabbatical to pursue extra
research or additional training as desired.

Career prospects

The job prospects for senior registrars and lecturers are not good at
present because only some of the retirement consultant vacancies are
being readvertised. Doctors who wish to make a career in this specialty
are strongly advised to contact the British Thoracic Society for guidance
on manpower numbers.

Rheumatology

Rheumatology is predominantly concerned with disorders of the musculoskeletal system, affecting people of any age, but many rheumatic diseases are multisystem disorders and a wide experience of general medicine is important. The scope of rheumatic diseases is such that, whilst many doctors specialise in rheumatology alone, others choose to be involved in fields such as immunology, general (internal) medicine or rehabilitation (disability) medicine.

The consultant's job

Most established consultant posts are in rheumatology alone, especially in southern England, but some districts seek a general physician with a special expertise in rheumatology or a rheumatologist with experience in rehabilitation. The latter may be sought less often as more specialist training in rehabilitation (disability) medicine develops. Whether to select a post offering single or dual accreditation should be given careful consideration before embarking on higher medical training.

Life-threatening crises and long-term care of patients with rheumatic disease require skilled management and close co-operation with colleagues in other disciplines and professions. Good organisation and teamwork are important. Much of the work is done in outpatient clinics and may be supported by clinical assistants rather than junior staff in training. As many doctors have little training in rheumatology, teaching skills and willingness to participate in postgraduate training are also valued.

Training requirements

Experience of research and study towards a higher degree is expected. There is still much to discover about the aetiology, pathogenesis and treatment of these chronic disabling diseases. Research may be clinical or laboratory based, covering such diverse fields as biochemistry, biomechanics, epidemiology, immunology, molecular biology and pharmacology. Academic units and other large rheumatology centres have specialist interests and will be able to advise on funding and supervision of work in their field. The British Society for Rheumatology (BSR) organises scientific meetings and basic and advanced educational courses. It continues to liaise closely with other bodies on manpower levels and training requirements. Trainee rheumatologists meet regularly and are represented on the BSR council and its subcommittees. There are also links with training in Europe.

Career prospects

The prospects in rheumatology have improved recently as senior registrar numbers have been reduced and the consultant grade slowly expands. There is scope for further expansion, as there are still districts with little or no rheumatological service. Rheumatologists may serve more than one district and it may be an advantage to have some training and experience in administration.